D1085683

Bella Ellwood-Clayton studied in Montreal, Canada, and completed a PhD on women's sexuality at the University of Melbourne, Australia. Her doctoral thesis was on the sex lives of women in the Philippines. In 2001 she filmed a documentary with *National Geographic* in the jungles of Sumatra, Indonesia. She writes columns on sex and relationships for several Australian newspapers and appears regularly on television and radio.

Some of the material in this book has been published previously: parts of Chapter 4 first appeared as an article in the journal *Philipinas* as 'Constructions of seduction: premarital sex in the Catholic Philippines' (2007) and as a feature article in *Cosmopolitan*'s pregnancy supplement as 'A Sensual Pregnancy' (Winter, 2009). Part of Chapter 6 first appeared in *The Canberra Times* as 'Love drugs are no cure for relationship problems' (28 June 2010). And parts of Chapters 1, 2, 4, 5, 6, 7 and 10 first appeared as columns in *Sunday Life* magazine between 2009 and 2011.

Acknowledgements

I would like to thank the women who told me their stories. I am grateful for the research assistance of Javiera Dastres and the support of Melbourne University's Writing Centre for Scholars and Researchers. Most of all, I would like to thank my husband, Stephen Turner: 'Love is the best kind of therapy.'

Sex Drive

In pursuit of female desire

Dr Bella Ellwood-Clayton,
sexual anthropologist

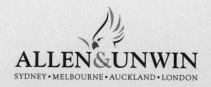

ALLEN&UNWIN
SYDNEY·MELBOURNE·AUCKLAND·LONDON

SOMERSET CO. LIBRARY
BRIDGEWATER. N.J. 0880?

The information in this book is intended as a guide only, and should not substitute medical care and advice. Always consult your doctor about medical advice in the first instance.

The photograph on p. 18 used by permission of the artist © Jamie McCartney. One of ten panels of 'The Great Wall of Vagina', 2011.

The poem on p. 160 is Jane Kenyon's 'Back', from *Collected Poems*. Copyright © 2005 by The Estate of Jane Kenyon. Reprinted with the permission of The Permissions Company, Inc. on behalf of Graywolf Press, Minneapolis, Minnesota, www.graywolfpress.org.

First published in 2012

Copyright © Bella Ellwood-Clayton 2012

All rights reserved. No part of this book may be reproduced or transmitted in any form or by any means, electronic or mechanical, including photocopying, recording or by any information storage and retrieval system, without prior permission in writing from the publisher. The Australian *Copyright Act 1968* (the Act) allows a maximum of one chapter or 10 per cent of this book, whichever is the greater, to be photocopied by any educational institution for its educational purposes provided that the educational institution (or body that administers it) has given a remuneration notice to Copyright Agency Limited (CAL) under the Act.

Allen & Unwin
Sydney, Melbourne, Auckland, London

83 Alexander Street
Crows Nest NSW 2065
Australia
Phone: (61 2) 8425 0100
Fax: (61 2) 9906 2218
Email: info@allenandunwin.com
Web: www.allenandunwin.com

Cataloguing-in-Publication details are available
from the National Library of Australia
www.trove.nla.gov.au

ISBN 978 1 74175 666 1

Internal design by Design by Committee
Index by Puddingburn
Set in 11/15.25 pt Sabon Pro by Bookhouse, Sydney
Printed and bound in Australia by Griffin Press

10 9 8 7 6 5 4 3 2 1

MIX
Paper from
responsible sources
FSC® C001695

The paper in this book is FSC® certified. FSC® promotes environmentally responsible, socially beneficial and economically viable management of the world's forests.

Contents

Introduction

The crisis in women's sexuality

It's the end of another long day and you've barely survived it. You stand at the mirror and brush your teeth, scrutinising the lines on your face. You wonder, as you open the little bottle, when you started using cream specifically for the under-eye region. Was that the point when you started ageing?

You crawl into bed and rest your body against your partner's solid form. Although he is also tired, his mouth finds your neck and his hands bring you closer. But you don't want the intimacy, the physical connection. You'd like to sleep, read your novel, or analyse why your co-worker is so mercurial. Besides, you don't feel the least bit sexy, and everybody knows that's the key to everything.

When it comes to women's priorities, is sex on top? A study discussed later in the book estimated that 43 per cent of American women are dissatisfied with sex.[1] A Canadian journal reported that 30–35 per cent of women experienced a lack of sexual desire.[2] Research in Germany found that once a woman is in a secure relationship her sex drive begins to plummet.[3]

Women are collectively not in the mood because inside our cerebral cortex, where arousal originates, there is a to-do list that is never-ending. And just when it looks like you've nailed all the tasks, another lot file in, obliterating any thought of sex.

Yet I find the shift in our priorities perplexing. Too busy for sex . . . but how is it that we still have enough time to soak our whites, get our shoes re-heeled and make pasta sauce?

In the beginning, it wasn't like this. In fact, there was nothing more important than our lover. In the beginning we yearned for him. We chose lovely outfits solely for him to unzip. We gave him back rubs, for goodness' sake.

But after moving in together or having babies, is it a fait accompli? Do we now rest on our romantic laurels?

I sometimes wonder what our partners would think of us if they were first meeting us now. The man you're with probably wouldn't decide to spend his life with a woman who didn't really feel like kissing him, considered sex a nuisance, and—as one study has shown, would rather he Hoover than hold her.[4] There are also costs arising from our sexual indifference, if infidelity and divorce rates are considered. But even worse is the loss of our own spirit and vitality.

We tell ourselves we are too tired, and perhaps we are. We are goddesses of multi-tasking. But what are we really trying to accomplish? A relationship that stays dynamic is like a well-tended plant—consistently nurtured and watered. It may be time to redirect some of the creative, dedicated energy we give our children, our dinner tables and our workplaces to the sensuality of our marriages and partnerships. When did sensuality slip off the list?

Sex is not simply two bodies coming together. Sex—the way we think about it, whether we desire it, how we go about getting it, and how we have it—is shaped by the culture we live in, by the time period we share, and by whether we inhabit a male or female body.

This book explores the female libido: what it is, how it works, why it becomes depleted, and ways we can increase it, if we wish.

Libido—most often defined as the drive associated with sexual energy—represents our desire for or interest in sexual union and pleasure. Our sex drive may involve fantasies, attraction to others, the seeking out of sexual activity, and increased genital sensitivity. Women's libidos are something of a mystery, because throughout history, female sexuality has been considered sinful. Our culture has never encouraged us to extend our sensuous arms to see what we can find, to see what we can taste. For many years, and still in many countries, our libido has been suppressed by religion. And most gods, it seems, cast a disapproving eye on sensual women—those who enjoy their desire, those who value pleasure.

The work of feminists in the 1960s has given women more choice. More money in their bank accounts, better contraception, higher education, and a wider dating pool.

From all walks of life, in all continents, women young and old are doing things differently from their mothers and their grandmothers. Including sex. They are finding sex online, with strangers, in second marriages . . . finding it for its own sake. But just as our shackles have loosened, new assaults have been launched.

It used to be the church that made us feel bad. Now advertising does the job. We may no longer feel as much sexual shame, but now we feel ugly. Our sexual expression has become less taboo because now money can be made from it. The new story has something to sell: it says sexual happiness can be bought.

This story tells us that our libido should be like liquid, flowing, abundant. Not only should we look desirable, we should also actively desire: *crave* sex, *initiate* sex, *relish* sex. As well, of course, as steering a career and raising glossy, articulate children.

And what of those relationships lacking in such carnality, or that don't match that impossible Hollywood portrait: the amalgamation of desire and familiarity, of passion and monogamy? They are decreed inferior, impotent. And the woman too fatigued for foreplay is labelled sexually dysfunctional. To counter their disinterest drugs are being trialled and marketed in hopes of discovering a 'pink Viagra'.

Recent studies confirm that lack of libido is the most common sexual problem in Western women. But how can that be, in the wake of the sexual revolution? Is 'low libido' itself a construct, a conspiracy of sorts against women?

Contemporary urban life is creating a mind–body disconnect in which women don't want sex because they don't *feel sexy.* Body image and childbirth can profoundly change the way women see themselves, just as parenting can rob their focus. Relationship, professional and personal problems also contribute to depression, and antidepressant medication often has a devastating effect on libido. Furthermore, ageing in a culture that glorifies youth renders the mature woman unappealing. To be 'natural' in our society is to be undesirable.

Women's libido is under real threat from the lives we lead, our relationship troubles and overburdened schedules, and from the wider forces of media and marketing. Expectations—what we *believe* we deserve, and what we *believe* our sexuality should be like—clash with the reality we find when we undress and lie naked in our bed.

A constellation of questions led to the birth of this book. They included: What do we really know about female libido? Do we have unrealistic expectations about our sex drive? Who defines what is normal and abnormal? Could 'low libido' in fact be the natural order of things?

This book has grown from the ground up, born from analysing hundreds of academic papers, and books about sexuality, reviewing statistics from around the globe, interviewing about ninety strangers and having many conversations with colleagues and friends.[5] When I started it, I was newly married. By the time I finished, I had two children.

I hope it helps you better understand and discover your own authentic sex drive.

1

Libido and the naked body

Instead of going to church for atonement, like many women my age living in secular cultures I head to the gym. For chemical salvation: the mood enhancement that comes with endorphin release. At first, I only went to yoga and Pilates classes. Here men and women held wide postures like prehistoric birds and made noises of wind through their throats. But after months of sun salutations, I desired a change. Enter high-cardio workouts. Body Pump, Body Combat, Body Attack. Like Army Special Forces, the women around me rose to each challenge. But as the weeks passed, I began to wonder why. Why had we ended up in this underworld of urban self-flagellation—to appease the gods of vanity? If exercise was the new religion, these were the fitnesscenti. But I wondered, in an age where sex is scarce, why were we getting dirty in the gym, but not in our beds?

Our desire to appear desirable exceeds desire itself

Being confronted by these pretty, dedicated gym junkies brought Naomi Wolf's 1991 book *The Beauty Myth* to mind.[1] How women look—or, more importantly, how we *think* we look—is still at the heart of much of our anxiety. The effects of this on our libido, our sexual vitality, are not to be underestimated.

Let's begin with a simple fact. Sex is far better for women when they feel sexy. Herein lies the rub: modern-day women rarely feel sexy. Far too much stands in the way. And often what turns women *on* and *off* is . . . themselves. Feeling good about the way we look is the best foreplay of all—but rather than seeking lust in someone else's eyes, we seek it in the mirror.

Women's sexual self-esteem often reflects how we judge our appearance against the current ideal. As a result, for many, the prerequistes of feeling sexy in Western culture leave most too tired, or perceivably lacking, to want sex.

The human body is not something we like to leave in its natural form. Across history and across cultures, we have adorned our bodies with flowers and jewellery, fabrics, dyes and make-up, tattoos and through scarification. We have altered our bodies, or mutilated them—binding our feet, lengthening our necks, corseting our ribs, and undergoing cosmetic surgery.

It is not new to suffer for beauty, and some theorists argue that preferences for youth and beauty are innate.[2] But in the past we generally adorned or altered our bodies to mark ourselves as members of our tribe or culture; beautifying acts were meaningfully ritualised. Our allegiance now, however, appears to be to the images we are fed by the media and the public validation we receive if we can match them, whether through exercise, make-up, dress, diet or cosmetic procedures.

Photography allowed images of the female body to be transmitted on a large scale.[3] Today we have constant access to 'beauty pornography', as Wolf puts it. The more widely images of the female body are distributed, the more deeply contemporary norms are imprinted on women's consciousness, leading to anxiety, bodily dissatisfaction and sexual ambivalence.

In previous eras, women had a better shot at meeting the ideal. They could henna their hands. They could tattoo their bodies. They could insert those African discs called *labrets* into their lips. But what happens when the beauty presented to women as ideal is physically unachievable?

Take Barbie. Most young girls in America, from the age of three upwards, own a Barbie doll. A study comparing body measurements of models, store mannequins and Barbie dolls found that: '[a] young woman randomly chosen from the reference population would have a 7 per cent chance of being as ectomorphic [slender] as a catwalk model, a 3 per cent chance of matching an international model, a 0.3 per cent chance of matching a shop mannequin, a 0.1 per cent chance of matching a 'supermodel', and no chance at all of matching Barbie'.[4] Talk about setting us up for a fall.

Women are more critical of their appearance than men are of theirs, and most women in Western cultures are dissatisfied with their bodies, which affects their sense of self and sexual identity. Feeling that they are naturally lacking, many women try to buy beauty. The British writer Susie Orbach says 'we have become enslaved not just to consumerism but to the body as our personal product which we must shape and reshape according to the dictates created in the market but felt individually'.[5]

Few of us are immune to the desire to upgrade ourselves. What with online shopping for miracle beauty potions and on-foot shopping for slimming clothes, famine dieting and other tasks of vanity, it's no wonder we have little time left for such primitive activities as coupling. And for the wealthy there is no end to the beauty candy in which one can indulge: teeth bleaching, lunchtime Botox, liposuction and stylists-come-analysts.

Despite the hours, money and emotion invested in beauty, fashion and exercise, few Western women feel they measure up. With advertising pushing a juvenile standard of beauty—unaged, unlined, undernourished yet over sexed—the competition is ruthless and impossible to trump. Cindy Crawford is quoted as saying, 'Even I don't look like Cindy Crawford in the morning.'

Increasingly women work—and pay—to fight the clock. Americans spend $28 billion a year on toiletries and beauty products.[6] Tweens (children aged 8–12) and teens constitute more than one-third of the personal-care market in the US.[7]

One study found that women in Britain spend an average of £3000 a year on beauty products and treatments, with 81 per cent wearing make-up every day; only 3 per cent said that they felt naturally beautiful.[8] Another British study found that women owned, on average, 86 different toiletries. Significantly, when asked how make-up made them feel, 73 per cent said they felt *sexier* and 53 per cent said they were more flirtatious. Only 10 per cent said they felt younger. The total cost of a lifetime's supply of beauty products and treatments was calculated to be £182,528.[9]

Wouldn't you think that we'd have better things to do? Looking good is important, of course. And it feels great—sometimes even euphoric—to have a new haircut, to buy strappy stilettos, to feel that some part of us is beautiful. But with millions of people starving, perhaps we should question our priorities. If we can't look like Angelina Jolie, perhaps we should act like her. Save the husband-snagging.

The Dalai Lama has said: 'External beauty—you can make . . . I think quite expensive. Some makes them look like [they] come from outer space. Therefore, I think inner beauty very important.'[10] A Russian archbishop says that if we devoted all the time we spend putting on make-up to prayer and repentance, 'true beauty would then shine forth from a woman's face'.[11]

Ironically, our hyper-focus on appearing gorgeous is having the opposite effect on how we feel inside. Rather than having sex, women simply want to *look* like they are having sex. Our desire to *appear* desirable exceeds anything to do with sexual desire itself.

We are too busy chasing beautiful to want to kiss beautifully. Too busy chasing the veneer of desirability, to desire. Yin and yang at play. The pursuit of appearing desirable negatively affects our engagement of desire. Our animal instincts have become inverted: time devoted to preening overrides time devoted to mating and sexual pleasure.

Enter the plastic age

We now submit to a new form of self-flagellation, cosmetic surgery, in hopes of matching the Hollywood ideal. According to the Australian National University's Rhian Parker cosmetic surgery evolved from reconstructive plastic surgery. This developed when syphilis was prevalent: the disease often caused a collapse of cartilage in the nose, which doctors reconstructed. After World War I, disfigured soldiers had plastic surgery so they could re-enter society. Gradually, women became aware of the transformative power of cosmetic surgery.

In 1926 a Parisian designer named Suzanne Geoffre, wanting to meet the boyish ideal of the era, underwent cosmetic surgery to have her calves made thinner.[12] Her surgeon screwed up, and Suzanne's leg had to be amputated. Suzanne sued. Amazingly, the surgeon's lawyers argued that because of the social importance of beauty, cosmetic surgery offered a necessary service. The courts sided with Suzanne, pronouncing that a surgeon should not perform a dangerous operation on a healthy body in the name of beauty. Now, of course, doing so is commonplace.

Cosmetic surgery is increasingly popular and socially acceptable. In Australia in 2010, $745.1 million was spent on plastic surgery procedures, while cosmetic procedures (including surgery) represented the fastest growing segment of the beauty industry, with an estimated 22.5 percent rise in expenditure in 2010–11, to $555 million.[13] Cosmetic procedures in the UK rose by 50 per cent in 2005 alone; women mostly desired breast implants, facelifts and eye surgery.[14]

About 12.5 million cosmetic surgery procedures—invasive and noninvasive—were performed in the US in 2009, up 69 per cent since 2000; 91 per cent of the procedures were performed on women.[15] Predictably, the most popular type of surgery was breast augmentation. There is also an increasing demand for gluteal implants, specifically to achieve a Jennifer Lopez bottom. Bootylicious.

The number of people under 18 having cosmetic surgery in the US has risen by 14 per cent since 2003.[16] American teenagers account for 4 per cent of the plastic surgery market, with 346,000 cosmetic procedures performed in 2004.[17] As with many US fads, other Western youth will likely mimic this trend. The most common operations performed on young Australians are breast augmentations, breast reductions, nose jobs and liposuction.[18]

Australian health sociologist Rhian Parker points to how in the past, cosmetic surgery was the realm of film stars and TV personalities, but it has now become the prerogative of 'ordinary women'. Indeed, ordinary women en masse are overidentifying with celebrities. According to Parker, women often turn to cosmetic procedures because they feel nature has taken something away from them through genetics, childbearing or ageing. The aim of cosmetic surgery, Parker says, is not just to change physical features but to deliver the *vision* women have of themselves. As such, women are 'enthralled by doctors who seem to magically use their power to make any woman "beautiful"'. These doctors, she writes, 'have become technicians of women's dreams'.[19]

Deciding to have cosmetic surgery may be a beneficial individual choice, as any viewer of *Extreme Makeover* or *Ten Years Younger in Ten Days* will attest. But this does not change the fact that our culture encourages the objectification of women's bodies and allows little room for variation in its standard of female beauty.

The body has become a site of renovation, a personal reconstruction project that supersedes biology. In the 21st century the successful body is lean and well cared for. This is no clearer than in TV shows such as *The Biggest Loser*, where the flabby and imperfect bodies of shamed participants are bared for all to see. As the American philosopher Alphonso Lingis writes: 'Our "body image" is not an image formed in the privacy of our own imagination: its visible, tangible and audible shape is held in the gaze and touch of others.'[20] Women's appraisal of their bodies, their beauty and their desirability is a product of the social gaze, as well as of their own inner gaze and self-surveillance.

Too fat to fuck

We can't talk about women's libido without addressing the weighty issue of women's weight. Like cosmetic surgery, dieting often stems from the desire to look 'better'—in other words, thinner and sexier.

An Australian study found that more than 92 per cent of women experience 'fat days', and one in five regularly starve themselves to lose weight. Just under half of the women surveyed said they felt fat every day, and 67 per cent were uncomfortable seeing their naked body. The main researcher Adrian Schembri said that women struggling with weight ritually check their bodies, with increasing anxiety.[21] If they are uncomfortable just spying their naked body, how uncomfortable must they be *using* their naked body—seducing, surrendering, unfolding?

The Australian Longitudinal Study on Women's Health has found that among women aged 18–22, 47.8 per cent have dieted to lose weight within the past year; startingly, 20.9 per cent of underweight women had also been dieting. And the mean age for the onset of dieting was 15.4 years.[22]

A number of studies have found that after looking at thin fashion models, people see their own bodies less favorably.

The increasing body-image worries of young women have coincided with a rising incidence of anxiety and depression. Australian researcher Richard Eckersley says our culture is 'eroding our sense of our worth and significance by parading before us people who are more powerful, more beautiful, more successful, more exciting.'[23]

From a very early age, girls are affected by images they see in the media. It's estimated that girls aged 11 to 14 are subjected to some 500 advertisements a day—most of which have been airbrushed. Our young female population is suffering. An Australian study of 8900 girls found eating disorders, smoking and laxative abuse rife among those aged 12 to 18. One girl in five starves herself or vomits to control her weight, and the number of girls who starve themselves has nearly doubled since 2000.[24]

According to an American study, the sexualisation of young girls and women undermines their confidence about their bodies, leading to self-image problems, shame and anxiety. These have in turn been linked with three of the most common mental health problems diagnosed in girls and women: eating disorders, low self-esteem, and depression or depressed mood; they also impair girls' ability to develop a healthy sexual self-image.[25] Through all forms of media—TV, music videos, magazines, video games, advertising campaigns—and the internet, young people are exposed to an adult world. In our hypersexed pop culture the message is simple: 'hotness' is the raison d'être. New York fashion writer Simon Doonan has given a name to the look many Western women, young and old, now work to emulate: 'porno chic'.[26]

Girls show less satisfaction with their physical appearance than do boys, starting as young as third grade.[27] The media also has a stronger influence on adolescent girls than adolescent boys. A four-year study of girls found that the peak onset of binge eating occurs at 16, and of purging at 18. It is no coincidence that these are the ages when young women become ultra-aware of their appearance.[28]

The Dutch ethnographer Harry Hoetink coined the term *somatic norm* to refer to the shared image of an ideal physical type, say Cameron Diaz. *Somatic distance*, on the other hand, conveys the degree of difference from that norm, say, ourselves. Women are experiencing somatic distance on a global scale leading, in part, to a collapse of female libido. As the author Susan Faludi observed: 'The beauty industry may seem the most superficial of the cultural institutions participating in the backlash, but its impact on women was, in many respects, the most intimately destructive—to both female bodies and minds'.[29]

How women feel about their bodies directly affects how they feel about sex. According to Australia's first large-scale national survey of sexual behaviour and attitudes, 35.9 per cent of women and 14.2 per cent of men worry during sex about whether they look attractive or not, and this negatively affects their sexual experience.[30]

If we are anxious about our appearance, how can we let go and open ourselves to the sensual realm and connect to our sexual centre? Religion tells us we should be sexless, popular culture tells us we should be nymphomaniacs, advertising tells us we need to be beautiful to have sex, and our partners, bless them, just pray to have sex once in a while.

Sasha, 28, lives in Melbourne, works in the fashion industry and has been with her boyfriend for eight years. Discussing her low libido, she says:

> At the moment I'd like to join the gym. I'm not obese—it's not bad, but I could lose 5 kilos. As I result I guess I don't feel comfortable getting undressed and being seductive when I don't feel comfortable inside myself . . . I'm sure some men are like 'I love you anyway', whereas my boyfriend actually suggests I go to the gym. Suppose I were to lose 5 kilos, I wonder if I'd be more in the mood?

When asked when she feels sexy, Sasha says, 'I feel sexy when I get dressed up, we go out, and other men pay attention to me.'

Lee, 39, works in retail, has a long-term boyfriend, and is a mother of two children in primary school. Of beauty she says:

> We all dream to be sexy and all the rest, but it's not at all achievable. When you do take your clothes off and are ready to be intimate, there's always that guarded sense

of carrying extra weight, or your boobs sagging, and I'm sure that doesn't help with the whole sex-drive thing.

Marla, a 25-year-old graduate student, says:

My weight definitely affects my sex life. A couple of years ago I was about 10 kilos heavier and I hated being touched. If a guy tried to touch my belly, squeeze my butt, or put an arm around my waist all I could think about was him feeling my fat.

These women are not alone in their discomfort in disrobing. For many women, perceptions about being overweight interfere with libido. A recent study found that 80 per cent of the Australian women surveyed felt too fat to want to make love. After rating their physical appearance, a quarter of the women said they considered their looks 'disgusting'. A quarter also said they'd prefer to eat live insects than walk naked in a lit room.[31]

We know that lots of men see women as objects of sexual pleasure. But what happens when women begin to see *themselves* this way too—as objects to be evaluated? According to researchers Barbara Fredrickson and Tomi-Ann Roberts, our culture's emphasis on women's beauty leads to *self-objectification*: the tendency for women to regard our physical self primarily in terms of appearance, and to adopt an observer's view of it:[32] *Body, pretty nice. Good hair. Face looks tired. Fairly decent tits.*

Given that men are the main consumers of sexualised imagery and expect potential romantic partners to be sexually appealing, it is believed that female self-objectification stems from the wish to appeal to romantic partners.[33] Self-objectification has been linked to body shame, anxiety and sexual self-consciousness in women.

The sex researchers William Masters and Virginia Johnson argued that sexual self-consciousness—which they termed *spectatoring*—undermines men and women's sexual responsiveness and satisfaction. Inspecting, monitoring and evaluating oneself from a third-person perspective while getting it on, rather than focusing on one's sensations or sexual partner, can increase performance fears and hinder sexual performance.[34] Similarly, David Barlow's model of sexual functioning suggests that the thoughts that arise from spectatoring interrupt sexual performance, and that impairments in sexual functioning are often the result of disruptions in the mental processing of erotic cues.[35] Preoccupation with our appearance makes it hard to relax, hard to focus on being aroused, and ultimately hard to experience sexual pleasure.

Self-consciousness may also reduce awareness of our own physiological arousal. Research shows that women are generally less attuned to their own physical states than men. For example, in the absence of contextual cues, women are less accurate in estimating their heartbeat, blood glucose levels and stomach contractions than men.[36] This also extends to the sexual arena: women's subjective and physiological experiences of arousal do not correlate as well as men's, with women underestimating their true levels of physical arousal,[37] possibly because of their greater sexual self-consciousness.

Studies confirm this mind–body disconnect: women's subjective sense of arousal correlates poorly with measured genital congestion. Basically a lot of studies were done where women were made to sit down and watch porn and asked throughout viewing how turned on they were. Beats jury duty. Although many said they had no, or very low arousal, their vagina told a different story. In other words, you might be turned on, you just don't know it. Even if you are physically aroused, this doesn't necessarily correspond to how you feel about it. Our brains are our true G-spot.

Although low body image is more prevalent among women, men are under increasing pressure to be lean, muscular and erect. As naked male bodies appear more frequently in women's magazines,[38] movies and other media, men too are becoming objects of the female public gaze.

Naomi Wolf uses the term 'beauty pornography' to describe the plethora of sexed images that we encounter. But rather than creating an environment of eroticism, the cumulative load of so many sexual come-ons only dulls women's libidos, for they prompt the devastating comparison: this is *me*, and this is *you*, and the space between is . . . vast. Nevertheless, plump-lipped, high-heeled model/vixens have come to represent sexuality to both men *and* women—making most of us feel rather unattractive, and therefore more easily exploited by mass marketers. As Wolf writes, 'Advertising aimed at women works by lowering our self-esteem. If it flatters our self-esteem it is not effective.'[39] It makes you think, doesn't it: if advertising got off our backs, we might just get onto ours.

But it is not only 'beauty pornography' that has led to mass female body anxiety. Sexual pornography plays a large role too.

In any given second, 28,258 internet users are viewing pornography and 372 internet users are typing adult terms into search engines. Every 39 minutes, a new pornographic video is created in the US.[40]

When once 'dirty pictures' could be found inscribed on cave walls, when once risqué centerfolds were tucked under the mattress, now all kinds of pornography can be accessed instantaneously on our laptops. We can go to any country and view any sex act. There are no borders. The effects of this pornography flood are yet to be fully understood, but it inarguably harms female libido. Women in pornography are typically young and often surgically altered. Even their labia look uncommonly similar—even, hairless and small.

Pornography has increased women's insecurity about their genitals. Artist Jamie McCartney's *The Great Wall of Vagina*—400 casts of real women's genitalia—allows viewers to glimpse the myriad shapes of the vulva.

Wearing make-up, undergoing cosmetic surgery or watching pornography—a common sex therapists' tool for couples—isn't innately harmful. But perhaps we should question the relationship between these and other factors that can undermine women's sexual sense of self, both individually and collectively.

In the advertising story the ageing woman's body is no longer beautiful. Nor is a mother's body, her breasts droopy, her belly repugnant. The message of advertising rarely changes: buy this product and you will feel happier. Beauty is consumable. In the 1980s feminists directed their critique at men's objectification of women, but now, most women are guilty of the same act: objectifying ourselves, and one another.

Beauty, sex and women are uncomfortable bedfellows. At one extreme are models trotting down the catwalk like emaciated long-haired ponies, representing a benchmark of female desirability. At the other extreme is us.

But what if we could find ways to feel sexy without comparing ourselves to others?

Doing things that make us feel 'in tune' can gift us with personal vitality. Being more conscious of what beauty pornography we bring into our home can give us more control over what images we compare. Cultivating dynamic projects can channel this drive away from body ambitions to ones that are more gratifying overall. Sensualising our daily life can provide an earthiness to our everyday affairs.

Leaving the house with our partner, having a glass (or three) of shiraz and a meal we didn't cook ourselves can help put us in the mood. But beyond this, real work is called for. Finding ways to feel sexually alive, alert and beautiful is up to us. We should not let advertisers dictate what makes us feel desirable, or what makes us feel desire. We must claim this territory back as something personal, private and individual, not simply a product of the market.

Let us applaud the woman who decides to leave the house today with a naked face, unpainted. The young Asian woman who tosses her skin-whitening cream into the wastebasket. The woman who, despite feeling overweight, opens the door to her husband stripped of clothes, ready to strip him of his.

We live in a makeover culture. According to the sociologist Anthony Elliot consumerism seduces by us offering instantaneous upgrades to our identity.[41] We have quicksilver desires. We make over our homes and our bodies—all in pursuit of perfection. DIY self-renovation projects are replacing DIY sex and meaningful relationships. In contemporary culture feeling erotically alive—full of vitality, zest, desire to touch, use your lips, express feeling through your body—has become overridden by a mind–body disconnect whereby women don't want sex because they don't *feel sexy*. Let us uproot this and redirect organic forms of sensuality into our daily lives.

Let's ask ourselves how else we could define our desirability, aside from the ways prescribed to us. Why does our desirability seem so much more important than our desire? Could we spend our time, money and energy, on something more rewarding than appearance?

I end this chapter with an anecdote. I once worked with *National Geographic* in the lush jungles of Sumatra, Indonesia. I was examining how physical appearance—particularly tattooing and body art—was experienced by the locals. By night the crew and I slept on the floor of the shaman's hut beneath a wreath of monkey skulls, and by day I documented the ways in which women adorned themselves—their use of flowers, beads and tattoos.

A few days in, I conducted a focus group discussion with the village women. We gathered together on a raised bamboo platform, above a noisy mêlée of roosters and pigs. And then I brought out a picture, an image of the West, which I was hoping would inspire stimulating research fodder. And there she was in her trademark red swimsuit, her blond Barbie doll hair like an iridescent halo. Aided by the translator, I

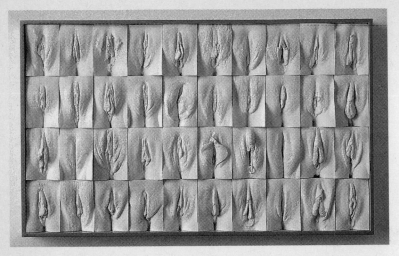

'The Great Wall of Vagina', a cast of four hundred real-life genitalia by Jamie McCartney, Brighton, UK.

pointed to the picture of Pamela Anderson and asked the most profound of anthropological questions: 'Do you think she's attractive?'

The women replied immediately. 'Of course she is beautiful,' they said. 'She is in a magazine.' I then asked the group if they liked the way they looked, or whether they would change anything about their bodies if they had could. They seemed confused. They looked at one another, shaking their heads. And then they said they would not change a thing, because they were healthy.

Oh, right . . . health.

In pursuit of looking 'perfect' if young, or 'young' if mature, Western women have become desensitised to the beauty of our body's functionality. We take for granted that we menstruate in mysterious synchrony with the moon. That our body can unfold and be rocked by orgasm. And that we can carry and give birth to a child. Instead of valuing these marvels, we demean our bodies. We demand more from them than they can naturally offer. We damn them not to age, and hate them when they do. Rather than looking down at our legs and thanking them for enabling us to walk, we curse the cellulite on our thighs. If our bodies were a friend or a lover, they would likely seek a more appreciative partner.

2

Desperately seeking libido

Men's Health magazine once called the bed the single greatest piece of exercise equipment ever invented.[1] Beats Stairmaster or Zumba surely. The pulse rate of an aroused person rises from about 70 to 150 beats per minute, similar to that of an athlete at maximum effort. Frequent sexual intercourse is associated with a lower risk of fatal coronary heart disease.[2] Australian researchers say that by ejaculating more than five times a week, men in their 20s can reduce their risk of prostate cancer by a third.[3] Frequent ejaculations—21 or more a month—have also been linked to lower prostate cancer risk in older men.[4] Indeed, sex, like carrots, is good for us. Regular sex has been claimed to have a host of physical and psychological benefits, from combating depression and boosting wellbeing and self-esteem, to reducing stress, thanks to the release of feel-good, pain-relieving endorphins in the brain. Sex and orgasms increase levels of the hormone oxytocin, which helps us bond and build trust, thereby improving intimacy. Oxytocin released during orgasm also promotes calmness and sleep, and can even help wounds heal faster.[5]

Having regular sex has been linked to higher levels of the antibody immunoglobulin A, which may boost the immune system and protect us from colds.[6] Sex also strengthens pelvic-floor muscles, lowering our risk of incontinence later in life, and boosts the production of testosterone, which leads to stronger bones and muscles.

If that doesn't sell you, the beauty effects might. Sweating during sex cleanses the pores, resulting in healthier skin. Screw L'Oréal. Depending how vigorous it is, sex can burn a lot of calories and tone a woman's pelvis, thighs, buttocks, arms and neck.

Sex also has the extraordinary ability to connect two people, to make them feel fused. To tackle high divorce rates, even the church advocates sex. For example, a Florida church challenged its married members to have sex every day for a month.[7]

Is sex the new antidepressant? Numerous studies have shown that couples who are satisfied with their relationship are generally more satisfied with their sexual life and sexual functioning. Canadian sex researcher Lori Brotto says, 'Ultimately we all just want to love and be loved. If people are sexually happier, they'll be happier in general.' She adds that sex is a mood enhancer, and although many women dread it at times, they usually feel better for it afterwards.

'So really there is an antidepressant-like quality in something that is nonmedical, very natural.'

For many women, libido is something we used to have. In the beginning of our relationship . . . when we were younger . . . when we weighed less . . . Then we may have felt that fire, the urgency to touch, bond, spread our legs and be filled. Libido was like a magic wand that could turn sex into something euphoric. Sexual thoughts would come, unannounced, jagged and warm. We dressed to be seductive, and used our bodies to seduce.

But for many women, libido 'just went away'. It might have been a gradual decline where sex slowly lost prominence in the scale of life priorities. It might have happened suddenly, after the birth of our first child. Either way, sexual vitality and interest became increasingly hard to summon, increasingly distant. And we were left feeling 'sexless'.

Libido, however, naturally fluctuates throughout our lifetime, and varies in strength from woman to woman. Even though some women's interest in sex is never very robust, the exception often occurs during *limerence*, the enchanted period of early love when sex is elevated to the realms of the divine. Limerence—the first months or years of a romance—this is when sexual desire peaks, not only because we are getting to know the most darling, amazing, delicious person on earth, but also because of the chemicals—dopamine, noradrenaline and testosterone—that surge through our bodies.

But what happens when there are children, and bills to pay, when we feel less physically desirable, when domesticity and boredom set in and those fabulous love chemicals are no longer zipping about? Some are left with companionate love that only occasionally hits the heights of sexual pleasure. But others are better able to tenure passion.

The lessening of our libido is in all likelihood a *natural* progression. Infatuation leads to pairing, which leads to less intensity as we rechannel sexual energy into other projects. But, there is a problem. We are living in a time when sex is the new gold and relationships that fall short are deemed not only inferior but sexually 'dysfunctional'.

Low libido certainly doesn't connote a sexual disorder. In fact, in the Victorian era, low libido was considered a virtue in women. But try telling that to hubby next time he complains. Of all the female sexual 'ailments', low libido is by far the most common. For many women, thinking about sex, desiring sex, initiating sex, languishing in sex is simply not part of regular life. Depending on the medical literature you read, the prevalence of low libido ranges from 25 to 43 per cent among American women.[8] The libido of ordinary women does not match the way it is depicted in film, television, music, women's literature and magazines, advertising campaigns and pornography. But, because we are so exposed to this media ideal, our partners and eventually even we ourselves can start to believe that this is what our sexuality should also be like. Whether distal—the body language of a model advertising handbags—or proximal—the x-rated files on your boyfriend's laptop—hyper-sexualised media represent women the same way: airbrushed, thin and horny. In the media story we should all have a flowing, abundant, liquid libido. Our lips should be perpetually glossed. We should be always in the mood and look as tantalising as we taste.

Is women's desire in the Western world at an all-time low? Could it be that despite feminists' efforts to gain sexual freedom we're just . . . not that into it?

The gap between the libido of ordinary women and the libido of women presented in the media leads to the pathologisation of female sexuality—where low libido is seen as a 'disease'. Women's first line of defence is often to launch beautification projects to try to appear *desirable*. The divergence between our über-sexed public space and our sexually muted private lives also sets up an opening for drug companies and their pharmaceutical cures (see Chapter 6).

What is low libido, and why does desire wane?

Libido refers to our sexual drive, but also our general vigour and enthusiasm. Low libido leads to reduced interest in sex and reduced creative expression of our sexuality. However, rather than dissipating altogether, our libido often gets funnelled from sex into other areas of our life: Our career can gobble that intense, heady focus. As can our homes, dinner tables and wardrobes. And most undoubtedly, a singular absorption with our children can supersede even the early, blossoming stage of limerence.

In other words, often it is not that our libido is low, but rather that our creative energy is being directed elsewhere, from seduction and carnality to more contained pursuits.

Hence the phenomenon of DINS, double income no sex, couples who are cashed up but sex poor. A surfeit of factors can influence the current of our sexual desire. Low libido relates to physical, psychological, interpersonal and wider cultural factors. It reflects our previous sexual history and whether we are single, newly in love, with a long-term partner, or a parent, and the extent of our satisfaction with these roles. It may reflect our body image, health, stress levels, hormones, emotional wellbeing, and expectations about sex and desire.

If your libido is not as high as you'd like it to be, here are some questions to explore. Is this low libido lifelong, or recently acquired? Are you or your partner bothered by it? Are you aware of its primary cause? Is your libido being funnelled into other areas of your life? Is your sexual self-esteem negatively affecting your libido? To what extent are you willing to boost your libido, or do competing demands or interests come first? And what would your ideal sexuality be like?

Molly, 31, lives in Vancouver, married, mother of a little girl

Tell me about your desire.

It would be really nice to be in the mood sometimes and actually initiate sex. But then I wonder, maybe I'm just not like that. I mean, once the newness of a relationship is over, when that excitement and mystery normalises, then you have irritations with your husband over not doing enough housework or spending enough time with our daughter, and it just really depletes any sex drive I might have had.

Do you think you'd see a doctor or healer about low libido?

I don't want to talk about it to anyone. I don't really believe in psychotherapy. I did once feel like acupuncture opened a sexual meridian or something. Afterwards I was working on the computer and suddenly felt like yay, I'm in the mood and went to look for my husband.

So for now will you just accept your level of desire as is?

Once my daughter's a bit older, once there's more time and sanity, then I'll be willing to look at other options. Right now I'll settle for lazy, infrequent sex at my husband's initiation.

Do you think your low levels of desire are only about being a mum?

I don't think so, although it's a big part of it.

Do you get upset about having a low sex drive?

I'm too tired to care. I know it's frustrating for my husband . . . Sometimes I feel like it's one aspect of my womanhood that I'm not in touch with and I feel like, yeah, that's part of me that hasn't been awakened yet and that is bothersome. And I do get a little envious of women who are way more in touch with sexuality and have healthy sexual hunger.

Where do you think your low sexual desire comes from?

Previous to my husband I haven't had healthy or passionate sexual experiences, and so when I first met my husband, I had to go through a lot of stuff. I was very uncomfortable in some positions, sometimes I started crying, there was a lot of healing in order. I feel like a lot has been put to rest, but at the same time I don't feel very confident in my sexuality and being a sexual being.

Would you take a drug to cure low libido?

I don't think so; I don't even take Tylenol [paracetamol]. It would be a really weighty decision for me.

A young Australian woman with a long-term boyfriend says:

I've come across women where sex is like a chore to put on the fridge beside mopping the floor. I'm not that bad. In general, I *do* want it, but I can't be bothered with everything that comes with initiating it, the effort involved . . . I guess I might be physically lazy. I'm happy to take it, but I can't be bothered climbing on top. I'm just like, come and get me. It's the only way I enjoy it, otherwise I'm not interested.

At the start of a relationship, that's all you want to do with the person. I think maybe I've had no interest in sex for five years, on and off. I go through phases. Also I find when I'm on a hormonal contraceptive, I really *don't* want it, so I'm not on them because I go pyscho and I don't want sex, so there's no point going on them.

Lee, 31, lives in Melbourne with her partner and is a mother of two children in primary school.

My sex drive has always been poor. It's almost like it's switched off. It doesn't feel normal. I don't feel like my whole body is engaged in sex. I feel like I have to work harder to get to the levels you need to reach to get enjoyment and it should be the opposite: the more you relax the more you're in the moment. I'm just not turned on.

Of the various factors that impinge upon our libido, there is often physical, psychological and sociocultural overlap.

Physical inhibitors: the uninterested body

A range of phyical factors can dampen our libido. These include conditions such as anaemia (common in women because of iron loss during periods), kidney failure, hypothyroidism (underactive thyroid gland) and diabetes, which may make arousal and orgasm difficult.[9] Hyperprolactinaemia—a rare disorder in which the pituitary gland is overactive—also diminishes libido, as can the use of some medications, including certain antidepressants. Ironically, the same device that enables us to have spontaneous sex—the contraceptive pill—if containing the hormone progestin, may lower libido for some women.[10] Alcohol or drug abuse can also alter sexual wellbeing and libido.

Some other conditions that can cause changes in female sexual desire include menopause, dyspareunia (painful sexual intercourse), infections such as thrush or urinary tract infections, and vaginismus—the involuntary clamping of the vaginal muscles, which makes penetration difficult, if not impossible. Pregnancy and breastfeeding also alter our hormone levels and object of focus.

The effects of hormones on female desire are covered in greater depth later, but we should note here that male sexual desire is also prone to the winds of change. Conditions that can cause a decline in male libido include age-related testosterone loss, impotence (the failure to achieve or sustain an erection sufficient for intercourse) and premature ejaculation.

Psychological inhibitors: the problematic mind

In the histories of women with low libido, a number of factors tend to recur. Many women reveal sex-negative family attitudes. Others have undergone traumatic experiences such as sexual harassment, molestation, abuse or assault.

Depression can cause lethargy, lack of motivation and withdrawal from activities including sex. Stress hormones can also reduce sexual desire and response. Work stress, financial stress and everyday worries draw us away from sensual living, and it is common for women to feel too tired for sex.

Lucille, 39, lives in Sydney, married, owns online retail business, mother of two daughters aged 2 and 4

Tell me about your libido.

It's pretty non-existent. It's very, very rare that I ever really think about doing it, and usually if I do think about it it's if I had a sexy dream. I'm more interested in sex when I'm asleep than when I'm awake.

I've even wondered, am I a lesbian or something, because I used to be more sexually active than most women. I've had lots of partners and stuff, and now it's just completely died.

Do you think your sexual desire has died off because of having young kids?

It isn't the kids. And it's not my husband either. I sometimes look at my husband and think yum, because he's really attractive . . . Even when we do have sex, it's fantastic. Maybe I've just gotten really lazy . . . I used to be a really active participant and now I can't be bothered . . . And I wish I could be. I feel bad for my husband; he never complains.

Could tiredness be affecting your sex drive?

Well, I *am* really tired, but I don't see that as an excuse. How long is an average sex session? It takes longer to drink a cup of coffee, really. I don't buy that. I definitely think there's something in the way. I don't use the too-tired excuse—I mean I do use it with my husband, but I don't really believe it.

How about sexual esteem—does the way you feel about your body affect your libido?

No. Look, I have changed since I met my husband. I've put on 20 kilos, but I'm not self-conscious with him, and he's the only man I haven't been really self-conscious in front of. I'm confident that he's attracted to me, because I know he never looks at me with a critical eye. When I was 20 kilos less, some men would say I was too fat.

Perhaps because you are so confident, you feel you don't need to work to keep his attention?

My last long-term partner always told me I was overweight. I think he had the power over me. But I have the power over my husband, so I make him work for it.

Additionally, sharing a home with parents—or worse yet, parents-in-law—has a way of dampening desire. And nothing dampens libido like a toddler, or domestic drudgery, which may explain why one survey found that the majority of women would prefer their husbands to Hoover rather than hold them.[11] On the other hand, over 30 per cent of women in a British survey claimed that cleaning gave them more satisfaction than sex![12]

For many women, emotional closeness is a prelude to sex. A lack of or decrease in sex drive can indicate ongoing relationship issues such as lack of communication or trust, unresolved conflicts or fighting, and poor communication of sexual needs or desires. Issues from our childhood or previous intimate relationships can also affect current feelings about sex and sexuality.

Although libido is usually strong during courtship, desire often dissipates. And were the discerning eye more observant during courtship, one would notice that even then desire was likely more in the hands of one than the other; that there was an unambiguous pursuer, and the one who responded. Initially, these inequitable libidos were part of what gave the relationship dynamic friction and oomph. But after limerence passes, we are no longer left with what the vision of first love promised.

If both parties are satisfied with a shift from romance to companionship, there's nothing much to worry about, continue planting your vegie patch, working on your golf swing or blog. But in most cases desire becomes unequal. Uneven. One wants more. The other is happy with less, or none at all. One longs, attempts, advances, the other thwarts, withdraws. A difference between two people's desire levels is referred to as 'desire discrepancy'. Dealing with mismatched sex drives is often difficult for a couple. Subterranean thoughts seep into the relationship . . . resentments, not feeling understood, not feeling desired . . . a sense that your true self is not being recognised . . . guilt that you're not able to satisfy her. Or him. Desire discrepancies can lead to conflicts, a greater lack of desire for sex, and eventually to adultery or separation.

It appears that many women make a great deal of effort to be seductive during the courtship and early relationship phases, then ease off as the relationship becomes more established. Some take their sexual life for granted and become sensually inattentive. At some point we may need to acknowledge that attitude can be a primary reason for low libido and that an effort is necessary to bring sex back.

Indeed, when it came to sex, many of the Australian interviewees used the expression that they 'couldn't be bothered'. One factor in some women's lowered sex drive is over-confidence of their partner's affections. Sure that their partner is loyal, they feel no need to use libido to maintain his interest. Because there is no gap to bridge, she makes no effort. With the chase over, she has nothing to prove.

It strikes me that we are absent of a script. Rom-Coms and women's literature seem to be all about *finding* love, not tending to it.

As we are single for longer before marriage, with many of us experimenting with different partners, we learn to be self-reliant, and our sexuality is tied up with our solo persona. Generally, the media focus on sex in terms of being single and in the quest for fulfillment, chasing and being chased. If sex is generally understood in the context of securing a partner, what happens next? How does love work when you have been together for years and years? What role does sex play within the dynamic of monogamy? The truth is that long-term monogamy and parenthood alter us, unsettle our previously built sexual personas. With the game itself changed, it's not just reappropriation or rechanneling of our energy that is called for but a *redefining* of our sexual selves.

Sociocultural inhibitors

Gender, religion, culture and the media shape our ideas about monogamy, premarital sex, non-reproductive sex, contraception, homosexuality, male and female sexual roles, what is good and bad sexual behaviour, and whether or not light bondage is a good way to spend an afternoon. Guilt and sexual shame can have a debilitating impact on libido—although taboos can also add a sexual charge. The contraception now widely available to Western women has had an enormous impact on our sexual freedom and creative sexual expression, but is seems to have contributed to the myth that our libido should be perpetually hot, and eager? In societies where women lack ready access to birth control, safe, legal abortion and sexual health checks, women are also more likely to associate sex with danger and to receive harsh punishments if they do not accord to local gender rules.

As we have seen, low sexual self-esteem negatively impacts female libido, as does the multiple roles of modern women: wife, career woman, mummy, domestic goddess, friend, and, of course, sex bomb. Culture colours all aspects of the above, shaping our sexual preferences, desires, fears and practices.

Interestingly, research shows that once in a secure relationship, a woman's sex drive begins to plummet.[13] An interview-based German study found that, four years into a relationship, less than half of 30-year-old women desired regular sex. After 20 years the rate dropped to 20 per cent. Men's libido, on the other hand, remained pretty constant. Oh how predictable.

Adopting an evolutionary approach to explain this, the lead author of the study argued that men's steady libido is designed to discourage female infidelity, whereas women's charged sex drive at the beginning of a relationship allows her to bond with a partner and, once this is established—think ring, babies, joint Facebook account—her sexual appetite can safely decline. Plus, if her interest in sex is only sporadic, the relative value of sex with her is heightened, further enticing the man she has partnered with. Human beings, after all, generally desire that which is not in infinite supply. Like the next iPhone.

The seemingly greater consistency of men's desire may be partly due to biology, but it also reflects gender norms. Since women and men are *expected* to have different libidos, they learn to experience desire differently. Women are raised to be careful and circumspect, to guard their virginity, to distrust their sexuality; men are taught something altogether different. (Watch any beer ad.) They are taught to be sexually curious, bold, to stalk sex, crave it, and then, in any given circumstance, consume it. This long history of women's sexuality being curtailed—limited and narrowly defined across cultures—has prevented us from knowing what female sexuality actually is in its natural form. Never encouraged to come into its own, to find its own form, female sexuality has remained mysterious, unresolved, an unknown.

At any rate, anthropology tells us that those who unite for reasons other than desire fare much better. Marrying for love is a relatively recent phenomenon. Anthropologists John Borneman and Laurie Hart write, 'The cult of romantic love in a companionate marriage is a recent innovation in the history of marriage. While romantic passion has existed in all societies, only in a few has this unstable emotion been elaborated and intensified culturally and considered the basis for the social institution of marriage.'[14] In the past, marriage was chiefly a financial affair, linked to status, property, inheritance, or in some places, the exchange rate of cows per bride. It certainly wasn't built on something as torrid and fleeting as passion.

If marriage was the stock market, a savvy investor would avoid any bonds associated with love. For the type of love that Westerners chase doesn't, by and large, last the distance. Arranged marriages, although they have their drawbacks, boast a global divorce rate of 4 per cent. In Australia, the US, and Canada it is around 40 per cent. What do Japan, China, Turkey, Sri Lanka, Pakistan, Bangladesh and India know that we don't?

Typically, an arranged marriage starts off with fewer expectations about what the other person—and love itself—will provide. Love in the arranged marriage tends to *unfold*, as each person gets to know, trust and rely on the other. Whereas mate choice for us, is similar to our experience of consumerism. Sociologist Zygmunt Bauman writes that 'consumer life favors lightness and speed; also the novelty and variety that lightness and speed are hoped to foster and expedite'.[15] Seeking instant gratification and armed with a list of desires to be fulfilled, we have expectations of love so grandiose they practically guarantee relationship seppuku. *I do*, until you disappoint me. *I do*, until someone better comes along. *I do*, until it gets too hard.

Modern love invites strife. On one hand we are told that Love is thrilling, all-important and sex is everywhere, and on the other hand we have what happens inside our four little walls.

Who measures up? No one. But advertising is built on creating a fantasy life that is just out of reach. Buy this, and you will be greater, better, happier, closer to perfect. And sexier. Few of us are immune to the lure.

Having discarded the various incarnations of god—within, without, animal or man—many have decided to take matters of their soul into their own hands. What guidance religion might have offered before—how to curb greed, not fancy our neighbor, and be happy with what we have—has been replaced by a remote control and voodoo pills to suck the sunshine back in. New purse, new car, new lover—buy it, runs the mantra, across the seas, deserts and aisles, and when it loses its gloss, trade it in.

In that climate, commitment and fidelity are often difficult to maintain as relationships become routine and sexually monotonous. In contrast, affairs often present a utopian edge, a chance to break-away from everyday domesticity.[16]

Over time, the unsatisfied sexual partner may look to another to fulfill their libido and do so covertly. Indeed throughout history and across cultures, the prerogative of many men was not to seek sexual satisfaction in long-term monogamy, but rather to have different women to cater to his different life desires: someone to care for him and his children, someone he can date and impress, and someone who will regularly suck his cock.

Sexual appetites

A couple's appetite for sex tends to fall over time. Relationships that begin in sexual intensity often shift into lower gear. For some, the new dynamic of companionship and trust can be just as fulfilling.

Australian sex therapist Rosie King believes there are distinct levels of sexual desire, and that most people with lifelong low libido are simply at the lower end of the normal range. She sees the scale of desire, from highest to lowest, as follows:

- **initiatory**—here you are motivated to have sex, look out for sexual opportunities and feel, in her words, 'horny'
- **receptive**—in the next level, you are receptive to sex and willing to engage if your partner initiates
- **available**—here you are prepared to have sex, but don't feel spontaneous lust
- **neutral**—your motivation to engage in sex is low
- **disinclined**—you experience no lust or interest in sexual activity.[17]

King writes:

> Concerns about sexual desire can be traced to society's dictate that the only normal level of sexual desire is initiatory. In reality, after limerence fades, the vast majority of women will never feel enough spontaneous sexual urge for them to make the first move and initiate sex. In the post-limerence period, most women will move back and forth between receptive and disinclined levels of desire.[18]

King adds that 'most women can't rely on high levels of libido to propel them to have sex. If women wait until they feel overcome by lust, lovemaking will rarely, if ever, happen.'[19]

Could this be true? Do most women in established relationships *almost never* feel enough spontaneous desire to make the first move?

It's interesting, isn't it. Women rarely feel 'spontaneous urges' to spend hours gruelling away in the gym, or have their bikini line waxed, yet we put enormous effort into such pursuits. We want to project ourselves as fully sexual beings, but when it comes to sex itself, we'd just as soon leave it as take it.

From newlyweds to sexless beds

In the course of a long-term relationship there are periods of transition when our sex life changes. Research has shown that frequency of sex declines over the duration of the relationship; as people age; as a result of life pressures; and after having children—the more children, and the younger they are, the greater the decline.

Sexual activity is hard to measure and examine. Many studies measure levels of activity only for the month previous to the interview or survey, probably because most people are more likely to accurately recall recent sexual activity. But of course the previous month isn't necessarily representative of someone's 'normal' sexual activity. They could have just been having a slow patch.

Unsurprisingly, people in stable, happy relationships tend to report a greater frequency of intercourse than those in strained or stressed ones.

Let's now look at some studies about sex for newlyweds, those in long-term relationships, those in same-sex relationships, and those in sexless relationships. Is all that starts off fiery destined to fizzle out?

A 2008 study analysed sexual expectations and satisfaction among 72 newlywed couples over a six-month period. It found that 61 per cent of husbands and 49 per cent of wives reported some decline in sexual satisfaction, and that 'those who experienced the highest satisfaction at the beginning of the marriage were most susceptible to declines in satisfaction over time.'[20]

It makes me think of that saying. If you were to put a marble in a jar every time you made love your first year of marriage, and then in your second year began to take a marble out every time, you'd never remove all the marbles from the jar.

In their 2009 meta-analysis of 25 studies, the researchers Bianca Acevedo and Arthur Aron[21] outlined the major theories of love. For example, Berscheid and Hatfield in 1969 proposed two major types of love: passionate love, defined as 'a state of intense longing for union with another' that is 'characterised by intrusive thinking, uncertainty, and mood swings'; and companionate love, 'the affection and tenderness we feel for those with whom our lives are deeply entwined', and which does not necessarily include sexual desire or attraction. Lee in 1977 identified six basic love styles: eros (romantic love), ludus (love that is played as a game or sport; conquest), storge (friendship love), pragma (love that is driven by the head, not the heart), mania (obsessive love), and agape (motherly love). Sternberg in 1986 suggested that love consists of three basic components—passion, intimacy and commitment—in different combinations: passionate love, infatuated love, fatuous love and so on. Berscheid in 1983 proposed an interruption model: temporary interruptions, such as separations, may ignite passionate love, including its obsessive component. (Think make-up sex.) Finally, Arthur and Elaine Aron's 1986 self-expansion model suggested there are natural mechanisms, such as shared participation in new and exciting activities, that can promote long-term romantic love. The authors of the meta-analysis concluded that romantic love can exist in long-term relationships and is strongly associated with relationship satisfaction, and that it doesn't necessarily run out or turn into companionate love. Obsession, on the other hand, negatively correlates with relationship satisfaction in the long term, but positively correlates with short-term relationships—hence all those glorious week-and-a-half relationships of our 20s.

Sexual satisfaction has been found to be related to physical aspects of sexuality (frequency of sex, orgasms), psychological aspects involving the couple (e.g. the woman's perspective of how close she is to her partner), socioeconomic factors (such family income), and demographic factors (age at marriage, educational level, number of children, religiosity, gender and ethnicity).

A study of 87 people in long-term heterosexual relationships (ages 23 to 61) found that those with greater relationship satisfaction also reported greater sexual satisfaction. Poor communicators reported decreases in both relationship and sexual satisfaction over the 18 months of the study.[22] Other research shows that husbands' and wives' ratings of satisfaction with their sex life were significantly related to the overall quality of their marital relationship.

A 2009 study looked at sexual desire and satisfaction in same-sex versus heterosexual relationships. Most of the 423 participants were white and well educated.[23] Those in same-sex relationships reported slightly higher levels of sexual desire, masturbation and fantasising about others. Generally, men reported somewhat more sexual desire than women. Women, however, had slightly higher levels of general sexual satisfaction across a wide range of non-orgasmic sexual practices.

After reviewing the research literature on lesbian sexuality, Margaret Nichols notes that although lesbian couples seem to have less sex than heterosexual couples, they spend more time on sex and include more nongenital acts, which results in more orgasms for both partners.[24]

Let's look at some other numbers. When it comes to sex, how often is often, and how often is not often enough?

A study of almost 3500 Americans aged 18–59 found that 54 per cent of men said they thought about sex every day or several times a day but 67 per cent of women said they thought about it only a few times a week or less. When it came to actually having sex, a third said they did it twice a week or more, one-third a few times a month, and one-third a few times a year or less.[25]

Another US study found the frequency of marital sex in 6785 respondents declined with age, from an average 11.7 times during the previous month for participants aged 19–24, to 2.4 times for participants aged 65–69.[26]

Survey findings from the 2011 five-country study (Brazil, Germany, Japan, Spain and the US) about sexual satisfaction among 1009 couples found that 64 per cent of men said they were sexually satisfied, 69 per cent of women said they were sexually satisfied and the average number of sex acts in the last four weeks was 5.74 times for men and 5.52 times for women. (Note: the study was supported by an 'independent investigator-initiated grant' from pharmaceutical company Bayer-Schering.)[27]

The condom maker Durex's 2006 Sexual Wellbeing Survey of 26,000 people in 26 countries,[28] via on-line questionnaires, gives us some interesting (if not necessarily representative) findings.

It found that 60 per cent of Australians, 55 per cent of Brits and 53 per cent of Americans had sex once a week, but fewer than half of respondents were sexually satisfied. The Japanese came out worst, with only 34 per cent having weekly sex and only 15 per cent satisfied. Greeks and Brazilians led the pack, with 87 percent and 82 percent having weekly sex, but only about half satisfied.

Respondents in Mexico, South Africa, Italy and Spain reported having the most orgasms (66 per cent), while those in China and Hong Kong came in last (24 per cent); globally, twice as many men as women regularly had orgasms. Nigerians spent the longest time per sex session (24 minutes), and Indians the least (13.2 minutes). Australians spent on average 17 minutes per sexual session, below the global average of 18.3 minutes.

If we consider the time we spend at the gym, reading magazines, web surfing, watching TV or shopping, it'd be a lot more than 17 minutes. And yet 40 per cent of Australians wanted more time alone with their partners, and 41 percent desired more romance and love. Spot the disconnect.

Let's look now at the way experts define 'sexless'. Sexless relationships, apparently, are those in which people have sex ten times a year—almost once a month—or less.[29] This seems extreme to me. Think about all those people who have been married for a decade or longer. All those people with kids. All those men and women going through manopause or menopause. If they are all able to have sex almost once a month, I say good on them.

A 2008 study focused on 77 people who desired sexual contact with their partner but were consistently rebuffed.[30] This involuntary celibacy affected the quality of their relationships, creating sexual dissatisfaction, feelings of frustration, depression and rejection, difficulty concentrating, and low self-esteem. Reasons for staying in sexless relationships included: other, non-sexual benefits; a lack of alternatives; social proscriptions against divorce, such as religious reasons, social image and commitment to the ideal of marriage; and other investments, such as children or economic stability. To cope with celibate relationships, participants invested energy elsewhere. Some sought therapy (either as couples or individually), yet all reported that this hadn't helped. Some gave up and no longer tried to initiate sexual contact, while others had other sexual outlets, namely masturbation or affairs.

From these studies we can conclude that people differ widely in how sex fits into their lives and the importance they place on its expression. What often starts off as heady and all-consuming can become a less central way of communicating. For many of us, this sexual demotion is the natural order of things.

Sexually inactive marriages tend to be viewed as 'abnormal' and stereotyped as troubled. However, it is possible for an inactive couple to be happy with their marriage as a whole, without sex defining its calibre. The hyper-focus on sexual frequency and the labelling of marriages that include sex ten times a year as 'sexless' reflects our obsession with sex as a measure of social worth. In our culture of sexual mania, it is dangerous to compare our sexuality to that of others, or to accept the current definitions of normal, abnormal, dysfunctional, healthy or sexless.

The problem with all this is that it is extremely difficult to measure 'low' or 'normal' desire, and the definition on which doctors are currently basing their diagnoses comes, as we shall see, from pharmaceutical company–funded research. Furthermore, what if low libido itself is a social construct, and isn't a problem at all, but rather falls within the 'normal' range of female desire?

Turning the tables, what if a strong, avid libido is the exception for women, not the rule?

3

Sexual prime

Men, it is believed, reach their sexual peak during late adolescence, while women come into their own at the ripe age of 35. What a cruel trick of nature to mismatch our desires so. With so much incongruence between men and women already, surely we could at least both want sex in the same decade. Maybe we are doomed to be forever sexually frustrated.

How is sexual peak measured? Does sexual *desire*, sexual *activity* or sexual *satisfaction* count most? It turns out that, as with most over-the-counter anti-cellulite creams, little scientific analysis has been conducted. Whether a woman's sexual desire peaks or plateaus at different times as a result of sex hormones is . . . unknown.

Sexual peak? A myth, says Lori Brotto, a Canadian psychologist specialising in female sexual arousal disorder (FSAD), who also heads an innovative sexual mindfulness program that helps women understand their libido. The last time I was in Vancouver I was able to interview Brotto.

Pregnant at the time, my 0.5 and I waddled our way over to the Starbucks on Tenth Avenue. There, the petite powerhouse explained the origins of the theory. Brotto told me:

> The myth comes from [pioneer sex researcher] Alfred Kinsey's data. The questions he asked were for different age groups. 'What is the maximum number of orgasms you have in a given week?' And he found that the 18-year-old men and 35- and 36-year-old women have the most frequent orgasms per week. And so that became translated into a man reaches sexual peak at 18, whereas a woman reaches her sexual peak at 36.
>
> But what the data doesn't reflect well is why are 18-year-old men having orgasms so frequently? They're masturbating all the time. And why are women at age 36 having the most frequent orgasms? Well, women—at least in 1953 when his book was published—were likely married, were likely in a stable relationship, and likely knew who they were. We know that orgasmic ability becomes more frequent with age and relationship stability.
>
> It gets translated into women are the horniest at 36, but it really doesn't reflect that at all. So there's some truth to those numbers, but you really need to understand how the question was asked.

Well that lays it out, so to speak. From Kinsey's work the concept of sexual prime was born. From one single study conducted half a century ago, a myth about the difference between male and female sexuality arose, was propagated, and became accepted as fact.

But orgasms peaking at age 36 is an interesting phenomenon. How many of these 36-year-old sexually blooming women in Kinsey's studies were *mothers*? Who knew piles of laundry were such an aphrodisiac. And why weren't the younger wives having just as much fun beneath the sheets? One key difference from today: most 36-year-old mothers in the 1950s had close-to-teenage children rather than demonic toddlers. Perhaps this sexual renaissance was the pay-off for marrying younger.

Women, we know, are most fertile in their early 20s. Being 35 or older places them at increased risk of infertility, miscarriage, and having babies with Down syndrome and other genetic disorders. So why would women be *more* orgasmic when they were becoming *less* fertile?

From an evolutionary perspective, maybe a thirty-something sexual peak helps maximise reproductive success. David Schmitt and his colleagues oversaw a number of studies which found that women in their early 30s, compared to women of other ages, showed higher levels of lustfulness, seductiveness and sexual activity.

The researchers came up with a number of possible explanations:

1) Could women between the ages of 30 and 34 (the average age of marriage) experience a peak simply because they are often newly married and in the 'honeymoon' stage of love?

2) If women are married by the age of 30, an early-30s alarm might trigger their desire to reproduce. If they

are not partnered, their 'biological clock' might awaken a desire for marriage and increase sexual desire.

3) Since research shows that women learn to masturbate more effectively around age 30, could the increase in sexual desire be a result of this new skill?

4) Might the peak serve to cement emotional bonds of commitment? As Schmitt writes, 'The early-30s sexual peak may serve as a mate retention technique for women. It allows women to keep their men from switching to a new and younger partner precisely at the time when a women's reproductive value is beginning its age-based decline.'[1]

Alicia Barr and her colleagues proposed that women probably don't need a raging sex drive when they are younger and more attractive because they are already in high demand. Plus, in that period it pays for them to be discriminating. As for young men, they are not as desirable yet in terms of social and financial power (abs aside), so it serves them to be super motivated sexually.[2]

According to researchers Robin Baker and Mark Bellis, the percentage of fertile ovulatory cycles peaks in a woman's early 30s and then drops steadily after age 35, with a massive decline after age 40.[3] As for hormones, oestrogen and progesterone levels are well maintained in healthy women until the perimenopause,[4] and levels fall when ovulation ceases at menopause.[5] Oestrogen has direct effects on genital blood flow, nerve function and vaginal lubrication[6] and is critical for the maintenance of vaginal tissues.[7]

Androgen levels peak around age 25 and start a gradual decline during the mid-30s[8] such that women in their 40s have about half the circulating levels of testosterone of women in their 20s.[9] While clinical studies have indicated that testosterone is important for sexual arousal,[10] it is not understood how it facilitates such a response.[11] Several studies have found that low testosterone is not linked to low desire or sexual function,[12] however an increasing number of studies report that age lessens women's sex drive and function. Richard Hayes and Lorraine Dennerstein reviewed the literature and concluded that women's sexual function starts to decline between the late 20s and late 30s. They also found that from the late 20s onwards, women experience reduced desire and sexual interest. Frequency of sex drops from our 20s and drops most sharply in our late 50s. Masturbation frequency increases to our early 20s, plateaus until our mid-40s and 50s, then declines.[13]

If we are to believe brat pack movies made in the 1980s men experience their sexual peak when they are teenagers. A man's level of testosterone is thought to peak at 18, and men have their greatest frequency of orgasms in their late teens and early 20s.[14] Perhaps Kinsey, who apparently had a wicked sense of humour, should get the last word on this topic: A doctor wrote that a man reached his sexual peak at age 48. When asked his opinion about this, Kinsey is said to have replied, 'My opinion would be that the doctor was 48.'[15] Touché.

Is it possible that when human evolved, a woman's reproductive success was enhanced by an early-30s sexual blossoming? Maybe. Such a peak would have come at the perfect time—maximising conceptive sex, predating a steep decline in fertility cycles and hormone levels, increasing mate retention and avoiding the genetic abnormalities, miscarriages and birth complications associated with having a child after the age of 35.

So there may be something to this mid-30s sexual peak for women after all . . . or is there?

Many sexperts dismiss the idea of a sexual peak altogether. The sociologist Pepper Schwartz has said, 'Sexual prime is a total myth . . . There is no physiological peak . . . no spike in hormones. No changes in the endocrine system. The whole notion is an artifact of the time.'[16] Fellow sociologists John and Janice Baldwin state there is no such thing as biological sex difference in terms of sexual peak.[17] After reviewing the literature and finding no definitive link between age and a peak in female sexual desire, other researchers conclude, 'Indeed, it remains largely unknown whether peaks in sexual desire exist at all.'[18] Clearly then, experts disagree on when a sexual peak occurs, but on whether it occurs at all.

One way we could attempt to resolve these questions would be through cross-cultural, longitudinal studies assessing frequency of sexual intercourse, levels of sexual desire and levels of satisfaction across the adult lifespan. Unfortunately, no such studies have been done.

I asked women aged between 36 and 71 living in Australia, Canada, the US and England to look back over their sex lives and reflect on a number of questions. Here they share their thoughts.

Do you think men reach their sexual peak in their late teens and women in their 30s? Was this the case for you?

I think men's needs are higher when they're younger. I think with women it depends on who they're with. If they're with the right partner then they're always at their peak.

Adela, 52, journalist, one son and one daughter, divorced, Melbourne

We are more hedonistic in our 20s, when it is more about what we look like, going to parties and having different sexual experiences. If you are single in your 30s, then you are perhaps more adventurous and confident just because of your age not because of anything hormonal going on.

Caitlin, 36, academic, married, Adelaide

I think men peak in their late 20s and women peak in their early 40s.

Angela, 53, publishing manager, three children, married, Adelaide

All I know is that sex gets better the older and more experienced you are.

Lillian, 55, bookseller, mother of one daughter, divorced, San Francisco

Personally, I would add 10 years to both peak suggestions.

Leanne, 50, accounting, mother of three daughters, dating again, Calgary

I think much of one's 'peak' has to do with expectations of satisfaction. Young men in their 20s climax easily, which isn't satisfying for their young female partners, so perhaps females seem to 'peak' later because we encounter or negotiate better sex with more experienced or better partners.

Joan, 58, lecturer, single, London

When asked about when libido peaks, many women brought up the factor of childrearing.

When you have kids your sexuality tends to diminish because you're breastfeeding, lack of sleep, et cetera. A woman needs a certain environment to relax and if you see that the kids are still awake then the mood changes. For me, my sexual peak was after my 30s. I had more control over my body and I knew what I wanted and I started to enjoy sex more than when I was in my 20s. It was after 35 . . . I've spoken to other women and it's the same conclusion that you know yourself more, so you're more secure within yourself, you know what you want, you don't need to prove anything, so that gives you some control. But sexuality has a lot to do with how you were brought up.

Carla, 48, hospitality, three children, separated, Melbourne

Both of us have enjoyed peak later (40s)—which is possible when children are older.

Jane, 56, financial counsellor, three children, married, Adelaide

I don't think that there is only one peak. Some women might be going through different episodes in their lives, different phases that might change things about their sexuality. Because we had our daughters young we didn't have time to think about

> ourselves as a couple. It was always about being a mother, a parent.
>
> Sally, 61, receptionist, two daughters, married, Melbourne

> I think sexual peak depends on when you have had children.
>
> Marie-Laure, 65, two sons, separated, Melbourne

Is there more than one type of sexual prime?

So far we've been looking at sexual peak in a quite limited way: does it exist, if so, when does it occur, and do men and women experience it differently? In a 2005 paper, Michael Wiederman, an American psychologist explored how sexual peaks seem in many ways to match men and women's life experiences. He hypothesises that this is a result of social norms, particularly the sexual double standard. In our society women are taught to stifle and guard their sexuality, whereas young men are encouraged to explore their sexuality through conquest. Inadvertently, this makes what young women are trying to protect—their chastity—more enticing to men. So it is no wonder, Wiederman says, that young men act more desirous.[19]

In 2002, Alicia Barr and her colleagues headed a number of studies of perceptions of gender differences in regard to sexual peak. They asked if shared ideas about sexual peak exist and whether sexual peak is defined in different ways for men and for women. They found that men and women both believed that women experience their peak later in life. Interestingly, definitions of female sexual peak related to concepts of sexual *satisfaction*, how good it was, whereas those of male sexual peak focused more on sexual *desire*, how muhc they wanted it. Also, after a seriously thorough review of the literature on sexuality and ageing, they concluded that rates of intercourse seem to be almost the same for both sexes across the adult lifespan and that women begin experiencing orgasm and masturbate most later in their lives.[20]

Back to our women interviewees. Here they share their thoughts on the differences between male and female sexuality.

What is the difference between male and female sexuality?

Men and women's sexuality is different. Because of the possibility of pregnancy, and women's stronger urge to reproduce.

Marie-Laure, 65, two sons, separated, Melbourne

Men want sex more often. Women need to be in the mood. What's that old adage? Men need a place; women need a reason. Having a conversation recently with women on how to spice up our sex life, we concluded a different man would be good. We grow tired of each other in long-term relationships. There is nothing like that first kiss that has you melting!

Caitlin, 36, academic, married, Adelaide

Older women are so busy juggling that the last thing on their mind is sex. Friends of mine who don't have these responsibilities seem to have the same libido as men if not more. So perhaps my answer is that they are pretty similar.

Pascal, 48, journalist, married, Melbourne

I do have an observation about men and sexual intercourse and it is thus: Given the invitation and the opportunity there are very few men who would knock back any chance for a random bonk! I think they are wired that way. This urge is probably most aggressive in their early years as the testosterone surges through them, and probably subsides with age, concurrent with the lowering testosterone levels. I have read somewhere that a 70-year-old man has the testosterone level of an 11-year-old boy—and that's not all that low really!

Iris, 67, artist, two sons, single, Melbourne

Men want to chase it, women want to enjoy it.

Wendy, 53, social worker, mother of three daughters, dating, Vancouver

Men's libido is always high—regardless of age, level of fatigue, stress etc., whereas women's libido ebbs and flows and is determined by many factors e.g. fatigue, emotional happiness, stress levels, state of relationship with partner etc.

Bronwyn, 43, dentistry, married, Vancouver

I think it's more to do with individual temperament, energy flow, way of being, that causes the differences in sex drive, not being male or female.

Lillian, 55, bookseller, one daughter, divorced, San Francisco

> Perhaps my friends are a randy lot, but we seem to equal our partners' libidos in spite of the well-documented complaints that men are always left wanting more.
>
> Joan, 58, lecturer, single, London

Passionate Marriage author David Schnarch believes there are two types of sexual peak that adults can experience: genital prime and sexual prime. The first peak is biological—when we are young and most fertile. The second is social—when we are mature, have more sexual experience and, one would hope, fewer sexual hang-ups. As Schnarch writes:

> Most textbooks on human sexuality, adolescent development, and family life teach that men reach their sexual prime before they even hit their twenties. Women supposedly reach their prime several years later . . . and therein lies our problem. Health-care providers make the same mistake as the rest of us: *We've confused genital prime with sexual prime'.*[21]

This, Schnarch believes, is a distortion. He writes, 'The speed with which your body responds is only one measure of sexual prime. Your sexual peak has a great deal to do with who you are as a person.'

His answer to the problem of sexual satisfaction is to put the beauty into sex. He believes profound, intimate sex is the terrain of the mature person, not the youthful amateur. Do you remember, he asks, being a 17-year-old boy, or having sex with one? Not exactly a Don Juan night to remember. While adolescence for males heralds the quickest erections and shortest refractory period between erections, this doesn't translate to much in terms of satisfaction, partner connection and sexual prowess.

Sexual prime, then, may be essentially about feeling comfortable with ourselves. It may reflect our sexual maturity, and our ability to turn a long-time lover on and make it feel like a first-time affair. Sexual prime may be something we can harness by relaxing in our bodies, stilling our mind, and, of course, looking in the mirror and liking what we see.

Schnarch concludes that 'a hormonal model is not an accurate framework for *human* sexual fulfilment',[22] and that sexual prime is most often reached in one's 40s . . . 50s . . . or (bless him) . . . 60s. Unfortunately, in his opinion, most people never reach their sexual prime. There's just too much psychological litter in the way.

Mirroring some of these ideas, British psychotherapist Michael Perring agrees that men may peak early, but that 'peak hormones don't necessarily mean peak sexual performance'.[23] Instead, he believes peak sexual performance is linked to environmental factors, such as the availability of partners. 'That's why men today are most active sexually from their late 20s, and still want to enjoy flings well into their 30s, when women their age are looking for a permanent relationship.' In his opinion, women's peak sexual activity now occurs in their 40s. 'It's not really about hormones. It's whether you've got the time, inclination and opportunity to focus on sex.'

Laura Berman refers to this second apex as the 'emotional' sexual prime.[23] The older woman, she believes, has a number of things going for her: 'You're socially secure. You're clear about who you are. You're more confident sexually, more assertive, less inhibited.'

Mmm, all this leads perfectly to the . . . cougars.

The cougar phenomenon

Witnessed on the streets, televisions and nightclubs of the West, the emergence of the 'cougar' is one recent phenomenon that lends anecdotal support to the notion of women enjoying a mid-life sexual peak. The term originated in 2001 in the bars of Vancouver. It was meant to mock women in their 40s seeking the company of men in their 20s. These women were considered desperate, 'out on the prowl'. The term went mainstream, denoting any older woman pursuing any younger man.

Why does female sexual assertion have to be linked to prowling for prey? Is the term 'cougar' an example of misogynistic male fantasy? Does its predatory tone demonstrate our cultural discomfort with older women's sexual exploration? Or could it be something altogether more positive?

Washington Post writers Monica Hesse and Ellen McCarthy write, 'There's a corresponding name for single males who prefer to date younger females . . . they're called men.'[24]

Age disparity in sexual relationships has been common throughout history and across cultures. But in previous times, it was almost always an older man with a younger woman. Now the reverse is increasingly visible. Men in their 20s (cubs) are dating yummy mummies who are 40 plus.

Yes, the term has often been played up in the media in a tacky way, and with a derogatory edge. Indeed, when it comes to gendered terms, women generally lose out: master–mistress, bachelor–spinster, wizard–witch, dog–bitch. Still, at least the sexuality of the older woman is now part of public dialogue.

So is the cougar phenomenon empowering or demeaning?

Valerie Gibson, author of *Cougar: A Guide for Older Women Dating Younger Men,* sees the cougar as part of 'the new breed of single, older women—confident, sophisticated, desirable and sexy. She knows exactly what she wants. What she wants is younger men and lots of great sex. What she doesn't want is children, cohabitation or commitment.'[26]

This is a far cry from times past. Traditionally the 40s is a time of losing confidence, perimenopause, life changes, and a sense of diminishment. Now in many ways, age is becoming irrelevant. It's about how you feel: 50 is the new 25.

Underlying the cougar phenomenon is the liberating idea of women of a certain age being free to conduct their sex lives as they see fit and embracing their sexuality on their own terms.

Following the TV show *Cougar Town,* in which former *Friends* actress Courteney Cox played a woman in her 40s named Jules, cougarism experienced a backlash. After the show aired, a number of critics called the cougar term a backward step for the women's movement. Of this, *Wall Street Journal* writer Nancy deWolf Smith wrote, 'This is the

21st century, where pole dancing passes for a statement of female liberation. So it should come as no surprise that Jules will search for self-esteem in frequent sex and the proof that she is still "hot".'[27] Judith Warner of the *New York Times* wrote, 'It's girls-gone-wild feminism for fortysomethings. It's ridiculous and belittling.'[28]

The cougar phenomenon has been gaining ground. A growing number of people are joining websites such as dateacougar.com. For a duration, in the US Carnival Cruise Lines ran 'cougar cruises'. Miss Cougar beauty contests are becoming more common around the world. Dating events for cougars are being held in Western cities. And for those who just want to watch, there was the 2009 reality-TV show *The Cougar*, by the producers of *The Bachelor*, where young men competed for the heart of an older woman.

We've come a long way, baby, from Mrs Robinson in *The Graduate*. The cougar phenomenon just goes to show how, when culture grants women education, financial independence and less pressure to adhere to religiosity, female libido takes new shape. And yet with all this hype and promotion and the 'discovery' of the well of older women's sexuality, are we also unintentionally creating even more expectations for ourselves? Not only should we be clever and financially savvy, not only should we produce pleasing organic meals, not only should our homes be stylish and our bodies neat and streamlined, but now we should also, come the later stage of life, have a rip-roaring libido.

But enough of science and social trends. Let's hear from women themselves.

Did you experience a sexual peak? When were you most attuned with your sexuality?

Now.

Marie-Laure, 65, two adult sons, separated, Melbourne

I performed like a dancing bear in my 20s . . . now I'm older and wiser, I know I don't have to. I love my husband deeply and there are so many other things to value in our relationship, like good wine and laughter. However, sex is imperative in a marriage: men need it like water.

Caitlin, 36, academic, married, Adelaide

I experienced several sexual peaks. Peaked first at 19. Second peak at 30. Third peak at 59.

Lyn, 63, counsellor, one daughter, dating again, Adelaide

My sexual peak was probably in my late 30s—unfortunately right when there were lots of babies around and not many opportunities to really follow up with my partner. It seems that the less time we have and the more tired we are the less sex we have—not rocket science—but we are much more inclined to go to bed and have a cuddle and really connect. God, I sound like such a nanna.

Maria, age 46, stay-at-home mum, four children, married, Melbourne

I have always been a career masturbater—one or more times per day—almost without fail, irrespective of whether I have been partnered or not. But now that I am postmenopausal I no longer have that driving urge. Did this urge reach a peak? Perhaps in my 40s, but it is difficult for me to say as I rather like orgasming and have always liked it.

Iris, 67, artist, two sons, single, Melbourne

I am much less attuned to my sexuality now because of the medication I am on. Methotrexate impedes libido.

Clare, 71, artist, married, Melbourne

I think as a woman my sex life has matured over time, meaning it has more depth. I have been married for the last 20 years to the same person. We have enjoyed a good sex life. There is no doubt that as we get older you do enjoy your sleep more. We have become very comfortable. Sessions are shorter and less often.

Julie, 55, manager, two children, married, Adelaide

I would suggest I was not sexually attuned until my 30s, and since then I continue to hone the attunement!

Wendy, 53, social worker, three daughters, dating, Vancouver

I was most attuned with my sexuality in my 40s. But I was in a 23-year relationship with a lovely man who was a completely inept lover until I was 40. I now live in London and the combination of menopause and men I find much less attractive has greatly affected my interest in sex with men. I still masturbate.

Joan, 58, lecturer, single, London

> Believe it or not I am experiencing a sexual peak now at the age of 62—but I am on HRT. I am very attuned to my sexuality at the moment because I have sexual opportunity. When married with two children there was really no opportunity for strong sexual expression and I think I just lost interest. I think it also depends on how self-expressive your lifestyle is—rather than biological age. I remember in my 20s feeling extremely strong sexual urges, but not so much in my 30s because my lifestyle was very restricted.
>
> Rose, 62, academic, two daughters, dating after being widowed, London

Several common themes emerge from the combined interviews. For many, sexuality diminished while they were caring for small children. The late 30s, however, seemed to resonate as a time when women could focus more on themselves—and their sensual life. For others menopause had a negative impact on desire. Some suggested that it was who they were with, not biology, that determined the scope of their sexual pleasure. Many women in their 40s, 50s or 60s said they were enjoying their sexual peak. Some believed that one can be 'peaking all along'—that female desire ebbs and flows throughout the life course, and that libido essentially relates to personal circumstances.

From our road trip so far, we can conclude that sexual prime cannot be reduced to hormonal and other reproductive factors. Our self-confidence, our romantic relationships, our lifestyles all have a part to play. Some speculate that there are two types of sexual peak: one driven by our bodies—our hormones and genitals; and one driven by our spirits—our maturity, our fluidity with life. Perhaps the two are intertwined in ways only we can discover for ourselves.

Since we cannot say definitively that women experience a later sexual peak than men, or if women even have a sexual peak at all, it is unrealistic to expect all women to have a similar sex drive. For those women who no longer care for sex, and for those who never really did, refuge may be found in our lack of ability to prove what is 'normal' when it comes to female sexual desire. If we don't know if sexual peak exists, if we can't define it, perhaps we can use this to free ourselves from comparing our sexuality to the sexuality of others and instead manifest our own sexual path.

The recent cougar phenomenon highlights the sexual vitality of the older woman. Perhaps for the first time in history, older women are being recognised for their innate sexuality.

We don't know if the stereotype of women reaching their sexual peak in their 30s helped bring about the cougar movement. But the rise in women's economic and political power means that new and dynamic roles now exist for the ageing woman. Finally, we are rewriting the script.

4

Motherfucker: merging eros and the maternal

All changes, even the most longed for, have their melancholy; for what we leave behind us is a part of ourselves; we must die to one life before we can enter another.

Anatole France

If you pick up any pregnancy book and want to read about sex and desire, you will invariably find a scattering of information in the section, 'Your Changing Relationship'. Women tell me that these few pages are painfully inadequate. What the books should *really* tell us is something we probably don't want to hear.

With the coming of new life, there is often a death of erotic life. The sexual couple may dissolve, either temporarily or, for some, permanently. Having children challenges a couple's sexual resilience. And diminished libido in the context of young children and family life may very well be the natural order of things. At least for women.

In this chapter we look at the relationship between eros and mothering. We explore changes in sex drive during pregnancy, birthing, and breastfeeding. Then we look at the effects of parenthood on marital satisfaction and the ways in which children can act as sensual rivals to a partner.

Pregnant eroticism

As we know from previous chapters, variations in libido between couples and among couples is customary; in fact, *having perfectly matched desires is altogether rare*. The physical, emotional, psychological and hormonal maelstrom of pregnancy further impacts upon sexual desire, and this can bring forth the unexpected. During the first trimester, owing to ailments such as nausea, vomiting, breast soreness, fatigue and the fear of hurting the baby, some women prefer to abstain. Fiona, 29, says, 'I felt sick all the time. I was probably throwing up five times a day for the first three months. With my sex drive, I was like, *Don't even touch me*. All I wanted to do was just sleep.'

One recent study found that 58 per cent of women experienced less desire than usual while pregnant, while 42 per cent had either the same or more desire (like a friend of mine who, during her first pregnancy, had 'the best sex of my whole damn life'). Indeed, many pregnant women experience a general low–high–low rollercoaster of sexual desire, based on their trimester.

Women can experience the second trimester as a time of sexual vigour. Rising oestrogen levels can result in heightened sexual sensitivity, and increased blood flow to the pelvic area can intensify sexual response.

During the third trimester and leading to labour, sex generally becomes less inviting. Katie, 34, remembers: 'Logistically sex is a lot harder. With the size it's hard to ignore the presence of the baby and sometimes the baby kicked during sex, which my partner found disconcerting. It takes you away from being in the moment and reminds you that there's a little person there.' For women who have sexual concerns during pregnancy, be aware that numerous studies have highlighted health professionals' lack of discussion about sexuality with women and their partners. In one study, fewer than one in three respondents reported that they had discussed sexual concerns with their doctors, with one third stating that they had broached the subject themselves.

Nevertheless, studies show that an active sex life during pregnancy is good for the pregnant woman and the relationship. But did you know that sex is also good for the baby? Orgasm releases endorphins that both mother and child can enjoy. The baby will feel a rush of happy hormones via the placenta and be soothed by the gentle contractions of the uterus. So instead of *eating* for two . . .

It is not only a woman's libido that changes during pregnancy; our partner's often changes also. In his book *Private Lies*, Frank Pittman argues that the transition period of couple to parenthood is a particularly high-risk time for male infidelity.[1] Charming. And a 2007 study reported that pregnancy was one of the factors that made husbands more likely to cheat, especially if they already reported being dissatisfied with their marriage. The authors hypothesise that women's declining interest through the course of pregnancy may contribute to marital tension and to their partner's desire for extramarital relations. The study authors suggested intervention programs to help men ease into parenthood.[2] Although it's rare for women to have affairs during pregnancy and in the first months postpartum, 4 to 28 per cent of fathers report starting a new or continuing a pre-existing extramarital relationship.[3]

Pregnancy often marks the beginning of a shift of a woman's affections from her partner to the newborn. Men, particularly, are often unaware about what offspring will mean in terms of their sex life and attention from their partner. Many men feel silently displaced and mistakenly think that it is only during pregnancy that their sex lives will suffer—not afterwards too.

Pregnancy alters our sexuality, our relationships and our bodies. Some women are shy about the attention pregnancy brings, some are proud, while others feel fat and unattractive.

Australian researcher Meredith Nash reports that pregnancy weight gain is one of the greatest sources of anxiety for women during their transition to motherhood. 'The fashion statements Hollywood mothers are setting are tight, small pregnancy bumps,' she notes, adding that these women 'usually opt to have their babies at eight months and have a caesarean to reduce the likelihood of gaining weight'. Nash also observes that 'Career women, who are in their late

30s and enjoy a fitness routine, find it difficult to not have control of their weight,' and that 'a lot of women are trying to put on the minimum amount of weight during pregnancy to avoid gaining weight after the birth of their child'.[4]

Indeed, in an era when beauty is equated with bony androgyny, feminist philosopher Iris Young writes: 'To the degree that a woman derives a sense of self-worth from looking "sexy" in the manner promoted by dominant cultural images, she may experience her pregnant body as being ugly and alien.'[5]

Young suggests that during pregnancy, women can experience a heightened sense of their own sensuality and a profound sense of self-love. 'The culture's separation of pregnancy and sexuality can liberate her from the sexually objectifying gaze that alienates and instrumentalises her when in a nonpregnant state.'[6]

Young refers to the relationship of pregnant women to their bodies as 'innocent narcissism'. Recalling her own pregnancy, she writes, 'As I undress in the morning and evening, I gaze in the mirror for long minutes, without stealth or vanity. I do not appraise myself, ask whether I look good enough for others, but like a child take pleasure in discovering new things in my body.'[7]

Young says the notion of a single 'self' dissolves as the pregnant woman

> . . . experiences her body as herself and not herself. Its inner movements belong to another being, yet they are not other, because her body boundaries shift and because her bodily self-location is focused on her trunk in addition

to her head. This split subject appears in the eroticism of pregnancy, in which the woman can experience an innocent narcissism fed by reflection of her repressed experience of her own mother's body. Pregnant existence entails, finally, a unique temporality of process and growth in which the woman can experience herself as a split between past and future.[8]

This magical time of being a self, a single entity, and growing another self that is both familiar and foreign, can mark an almost mystical change in a woman's life.

There is a lesson here for us, even beyond the realm of pregnancy. We must learn how to marvel at our wondrous body, ever changing, and to experience it fully, without appraisal. By doing so we will be closer to having a truly dynamic and whole sense of sexual self.

Birth

Historically, giving birth has been understood as a natural female rite of passage, with women assisting other women. Some have called birthing transcendent and explored the erotic sensations experienced by women giving birth. The American poet and feminist Adrienne Rich writes:

> Childbirth is (or may be) one aspect of the entire process of a woman's life, beginning with her own expulsion from her mother's body, her own sensual sucking or being held by a woman, through her earliest sensations of clitoral eroticism and the vulva as a source of pleasure, her growing sense of her own body and its strengths, her masturbation, her menses, her physical relationship to nature and to other

human beings, her first and subsequent orgasmic experiences with another's body, her conception, pregnancy, to the moment of first holding her child. But that moment is still only a point in the process if we conceive it not according to patriarchal ideas of childbirth as a kind of production, but as part of female experience.[9]

Rich even claims that if they give birth without obstetric injury, women have 'biologically increased capacity for genital pleasure'.[10] Anthropologist Sheila Kitzinger believes pregnancy and the experience of childbirth can even open a door to eroticism, and that the intensity of labour and drama of delivery may help women later let go during sexual activity.[11]

Unlike previous generations, most of us have never witnessed a birth or aided in one. Birth is now treated as a medical condition, for hospitals, not homes.

It is common these days to have one's husband or partner present during the delivery of a baby. In fact, choosing *not* to have your partner in the delivery room is now akin to smoking in public whilst pregnant. Edit that, unless French.

Indeed birth—at least Western, moneyed birth—has become a joint affair. But this is an entirely new phenomenon. It was not the case for my mother. Nor for her mother, or my great-grandmother before her. Historically there was men's business, there was women's business, and that was that . . . until the 1970s. Besides burning their bras and exploring their vulvas, women wanted something else. They wanted male contribution. Blink and we're in hospital beds with screaming woman, man at her side: a dove pair.

Nuclear set-ups have created one of the biggest social shifts in human history. Instead of living in extended family and clan networks, many of us now live in cities with a wife/husband/partner and a mortgage, families often continents away, soothed by the cyber bandaids of Skype and Facebook.

The pregnant woman, her belly bellowing, the birthing woman, her body pushing, and the new mother, with a small infant needing milk, stand relatively alone. Who do they rely upon for support? Usually, the weight rests upon her nuclear construction: their partner, a scattering of often transient friends and themselves. This lack of helping hands leads directly into the death of a new mother's libido. The danger is that the *mort*, the deadening of sex drive, solidifies and becomes her nominal identity as mother. Exhaustion and seduction were never close bedfellows.

This couple-centered paradigm has placed unexpected pressure on the relationship. In times past, a woman had her mother, aunts and sisters to help carry some of the domestic burden, both before and after the birth, and thus allow her time to be with her partner unbridled by child. Now, with man and woman having to play so many roles for each other, they are left lacking and can slowly become sexually diluted to one another.

During the lead-up to my first child's birth, my husband sought the opinion of other fathers about their experience of their own children's birth. (His research earned him home rewards.) Almost unanimously the sentiment was, 'It's a miracle, but stay away from the business end.' The business end . . . the nether regions, where gore and danger lurk.

Yes, birth is amazing, *the* crowning miracle. But is it possible that we underestimate the effects on our partners of witnessing birth? Certainly there is an abundance of literature pertaining to vaginal trauma during birth that women experience, which consequently influences how they feel about their bodies, sex and desire. Yet for men there remains a silence around the negative aspects of birth participation, around the disturbance many men must feel seeing their lover's vagina—previously a place of refuge, merging and pleasure—now tearing, bleeding and leaking. Particularly so when the delivery is complicated.

In our increasingly medicalised culture, where natural events are treated as medical conditions, excessive fear about the pain of childbirth is becoming commonplace. It even has a name: tokophobia. Some Western women face their fears by choosing a water birth accompanied by hypnotherapy and African drumming on their iPod. Others increasingly opt for a caesarean delivery. During the 1960s in Australia, only 4 per cent of women had caesareans. Now 29 per cent do. In many countries, researchers have found higher caesarean rates among privately insured women who, ironically, are at the lowest risk of birth complications.[12]

Interestingly, a 1997 study asked British obstetricians whether they themselves or their partners would undergo elective caesareans rather than a vaginal delivery; 17 per cent said they would, owing to fear of long-term anal sphincter damage or stress incontinence (100 per cent of respondents), fear of perineal damage (88 per cent), concern about the long-term effect of vaginal delivery on sexual function (58 per cent), fear of damage to the baby (39 per cent), and desire for a timed delivery (27 per cent).[13] Victoria Beckham was dubbed *'too posh to push'* for choosing to have a designer C-section without any compelling medical reason. Beckham is one of a number of celebs reportedly having early caesareans to avoid the final month of . . . abdominal stretching.

Indeed, while women are increasingly concerned about the impact a baby will have on their body shape, they're also concerned about the shape of something a little more private: what I call the 'vanity vagina'. Mandy, a young colleague of mine, comments:

> Most of my friends say that they are going to have c-sections when the time comes for us to stop making cocktails and start making babies. They don't want the 'sausage in the grand canyon' sex afterwards. A couple of the girls said they want to have lipo, tummy tucks and boob jobs with their caesareans. I hope this will change as we grow up a bit. It's nice to look good but, I don't know, I don't think body should come before baby. And hubby should love you, baby weight or not.

One woman told me that her friend took part in a chat-room conversation on 'c-section for a tight vagina'. This desire comes up time and time again in studies about childbirth, only worded more neutrally. C-sections are desired to preserve 'sexual function', 'vaginal tone' or 'vaginal tonicity', 'to keep sexual performance intact', or to maintain 'aesthetics and sexual pleasure'.

In fact, at three to four months postpartum, women's vaginas are mostly unchanged, although vaginal tension is slacker in about 20 per cent.[14] Nevertheless, fears about the vagina remaining loose after delivery appear common. Amazingly, it appears that the c-section, originally an emergency procedure, has become routine, and is often done in pursuit of the vanity vagina proving even our birth canal isn't immune to commercialism. Moreover, it seems that having a desirable-looking vagina is much more important for many women than their own *desiring*, reflecting a deep discomfort with their naked body.

For the new mother, birth isn't just a beginning but a conclusion as well. As Iris Young writes:

> It signals the close of a process that has been undergoing for nine months, the leaving of this unique body she has moved through, always surprising her in its boundary changes and inner kicks. Especially if this is her first child she experiences the birth as a transition to a new self that she may both desire and fear.[11]

Almost inevitable during the early years of childrearing is the demise of a mother's self-identity as carefree, rapturous lover. New demands on an already busy life limit time and space for sensuality and for the couple. As such, the sexual self can become lost at sea. After reviewing the literature, pregnancy expert Kirsten von Sydow concluded that 'the majority of couples have sexual problems immediately postpartum, and at least one-third of couples develop serious, long-lasting, psychosexual disturbances after the birth of their first baby'.[16]

Throughout history I doubt that most new mothers spent much time making love. They had other pressing things to attend to. Often, husbands found sexual pleasure elsewhere *and* were not condemned for doing so. Yet today we desire: excitement within familiarity, passion within monogamy, and sexuality within family. Many people trying to realise these expectations in their everyday lives find their relationship ultimately lacking.

Postnatal depression

A woman in her mid-30s told me she experienced depression after her son was born and that this alienated her partner. 'He was like, *What's the matter with you, our life is brilliant, we have a baby, why are you being like this?* It seems to me that there was nothing to do to shift the anxiety and stress. You know everything is good on the surface, that's why your partner can't comprehend it. Sexually I was completely mute . . . I didn't have a sexual pulse in my body.'

Although postnatal depression is not our focus here, let us look briefly at its occurrence and risk factors.

Postnatal depression may develop suddenly or gradually between one month and one year after the birth of a baby. It affects almost 16 per cent of new mothers in Australia.[17]

Physical, biological and psychological factors include: a history of depression and/or anxiety, a stressful pregnancy, depression during the current pregnancy, a family history of mental disorders, past abuse, a difficult labour, being single, problems with the baby's health, and issues associated with breastfeeding.[18]

Symptoms may include mood changes (e.g., feeling anxious, depressed, tearful), obsessional thoughts or thought changes (e.g., guilt, feeling hopeless), behaviour changes (e.g., lack of motivation), physical changes (e.g., lacking energy, poor concentration), finding it hard to love the baby, feeling angry, and having problems with loved ones.

A 2009 study of depression among Chinese and Caucasian women found that they experienced a discrepancy between the reality of motherhood and how it is portrayed in the media:

> The Australian women described the cultural image of motherhood—the superwoman myth crossed with the image of the Mother-Madonna—and said that Madonna-style motherhood as an ideal was relentless . . . One said: 'Those lovely commercial advertisements, which exist on television, in the newspapers, and in books and magazines and are for baby soap or shampoo, diapers, baby food, or baby clothes. They portray a smiling baby with a serene mother, and they contain wonderful soft fuzziness.'[19]

Guilt was the predominant emotion underlying the women's depression. They felt guilty for not being able to take proper care of the baby and the household. This sense of guilt was a barrier to reaching out for help and made the women feel that they had no right to care for themselves. One said: 'I constantly felt guilty because . . . as a mum I should be aware of all that sort of stuff [cleaning the house] and I should be looking after all that stuff [laundry, dishes, etc].'[20]

Women suffering from postnatal depression should contact their local doctor, visit www.beyondblue.org.au or call the Beyond Blue info line, 1300 224 636.

Mummy tummy

A friend of mine's mother is encouraging her to have children while she's still 'young'. Not because she might have more energy dealing with the terrible twos, totalitarian threes and frightening fours. Not because fertility falls after age 35. No, my friend's mother wants her to have children as soon as possible so she can get her figure back. Supposedly, if a woman reproduces early it's more likely she will bounce back into shape. For those of us over 30, the only things likely to bounce are droopy breasts and mummy tummies.

On warm days, you'll find my son and me at the local outdoor pool. While we wade in the baby pool, I look across to the other side of the swimming centre. Here women who have obviously spent a lot time in the gym flutter about in the water, stride around as though on a catwalk, or lay exposing their little derrières to the sun. And almost all of them wear bikinis. The women around me, applying sunscreen to squealing toddlers, have on another costume altogether: the one-piece or T-shirt ensemble.

Women are rarely prepared for the shape of motherhood. British doctor Lorraine Ishak believes that only one in ten women can expect to revert to their pre-pregnancy shape and size. 'Recovery', in her opinion, isn't so much about age—although loss of skin elasticity is part of the ageing process—but rather about genetics and body shape. Regardless of diet and exercise, Ishak says, weight gain, slackening breasts, loose stomach skin and stretch marks are inescapable badges of motherhood.[21] But she would say that, wouldn't she, being a plastic surgeon?

On a US forum about body image post-baby, one mum wrote: 'Frankly I'm beyond caring anymore. Yeah, I could lose 20 lb and plan to lose at least 10 of that by Easter, but it's too much work to worry about it anymore! That extra baby weight is here to stay. Too bad the "baby" is 8½ years old!' Another mum's comment was, 'Well, childbirth turned me into a marsupial. I could smuggle contraband with my extra pouch.'[22]

Mummy tummy anxiety is big business. Some mums luck out and regain their figure, some accept what they have and move on, some work out and try to resculpt, while others turn to surgery for a 'mummy tuck'—a triple operation combining breast lift, tummy tuck and liposuction.

And then there are women like Marla (35, married, mother of young twins): 'Before you have a baby, it's much more about what you look like in the world. My body was more sexual or something—but also more superficial. But now, because your body has grown a baby and been through this phenomenal process, now there's more substance to it.'

Myself, for now I'm going to stick to my side of the pool and just concentrate on playing pass-the-ball with my son.

Eros and the breastfeeding mother

No doubt about it, breastfeeding is sensual.

Any woman who has held a hungry baby in her arms and heard its cry for milk, or watched the satisfaction on her baby's face as he engulfs her nipple, or seen her child finish a feed, head slackening, eyes rolling backwards as he enters oblivion, knows this secret.

Social anthropologist Sheila Kitzinger has described breastfeeding as 'a psychosexual process'[23] which 'involves a flow of sexual energy through a woman's whole body'.[24] Breastfeeding, like sex, is about desire, union and satiation. To a baby, bliss is milk, and to a mother, bliss is often being the one with the magic elixir.

According to Alison Bartlette's book *Breastwork*, the eroticism of breastfeeding was widely discussed in the maternal literature in the 1960s and 1970s.[25] Indeed, the landmark 1966 Masters and Johnson study of human sexuality reported that 'women often become sexually aroused during nursing; some women have orgasms in this fashion'.[26] Yet now, the recognised hormonal links between orgasm, childbirth and lactation are rarely mentioned. According to Kirsten von Sydow, one-third to one-half of mothers describe breastfeeding as erotic, and one-quarter have associated feelings of guilt.[27]

But certainly not all women feel sensual while breastfeeding. Plenty tell me they 'feel like a cow'. An Irish woman in my mothers' group wouldn't breastfeed in public. When I asked why, she said, 'Truthfully, my wee girl is a bit savage when nursing. I wouldn't dare feed in public because she'd probably make a spectacle of herself.'

Nevertheless, many do find breastfeeding somewhat erotic. A study in Italy in the early 1980s found that the erotic potential of breastfeeding is often downplayed because it threatens to disrupt the 'only erotic feeling allowed to the mother in a patriarchal society'.[28] The feminist Germaine Greer writes, 'In modern consumer society, the attack on mother–child eroticism took its total form; breastfeeding was proscribed and the breasts reserved for the husband's fetishistic delectation.'[29]

We are taught not to acknowledge our maternal sensuality, but to censure it or keep silent. Voicing the pleasure involved in childrearing can be a volatile issue, as the following case indicates. In the US in the early 1990s, a woman had her child taken into protective custody for almost a year because she rang a volunteer helpline to discuss her feelings of mild arousal when breastfeeding her two-year-old daughter. She hoped to be put through to a breastfeeding support group. However, because of the 'sexual nature' of the call, it was forwarded to a rape crisis centre, which notified the police, suspecting child abuse. She was charged with 'sexual abuse in the first degree'—specifically 'mouth to breast contact' and 'hand to breast contact', though the charge was eventually dropped.[30]

It's no wonder that breastfeeding brings pleasure. The chemicals released in our brain during breastfeeding are the same ones released during lovemaking.[31] Suckling stimulates the nerve endings in the nipple and areola, signalling the pituitary gland to release the hormones prolactin and oxytocin. Prolactin causes the alveoli to take nutrients from the blood supply and turn them into breast milk. Oxytocin, also called the hormone of love, causes the cells around the alveoli to contract and eject milk down the milk ducts, a reflex called 'let-down'. Hanging out with friends, cuddling a loved one, having sex and birthing can also induce oxytocin release.

It appears that oxytocin rushes arising from breastfeeding, and the sensuality of caring for a child, dampen desire towards our partners, and that prolactin, which decreases sexual desire, also deters us from resuming a sexual relationship. In fact, mothers who breastfeed longest resume intercourse later than other mothers, have slightly less sexual desire and experience less enjoyment from intercourse.[32] Our chemical make-up, then, more or less supports sexual abstinence during the breastfeeding period. There is speculation

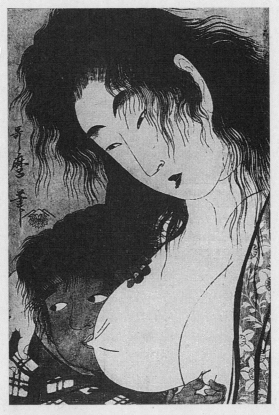

Yama-Uba and Kintaro by Utamaro.

that for some, the return of fertility also marks a return of sexual desire.

It is often hard to transition from soft and nurturing nursing mother to sex vixen; it just seems too incongruent. While a small minority of women experience high libido during the breastfeeding period, and heightened feelings of tenderness can spill over to the sexual relationship, the sensation of being 'touched out' is common for many women. Having to service the newborn almost continuously leaves many women feeling that their partner's desire to be intimate is just another pressure, another demand.

A new mother's sensual focus turns to her baby, and unless checked can remain the spotlight of her desire for years to come. And although we may be designed this way, our cultural expectations of marriage mean that this shift can lead to discord.

During the nursing period, many men feel excluded. Their partner's breasts can seem 'off limits' and taboo, and her sexuality can seem like lost territory.

For many women, the relationship with their child is their first experience of being awed by love. Since a baby changes and develops almost perceptibly by the hour, this fixation on the child can easily trump all else. Women who are lonely or in romantically disenchanted relationships may be in peril of developing overzealous intimacy with their offspring.

Love for her child is often greater and deeper than a woman has ever experienced. This is not what she expected, nor is it something she discusses, or necessarily even acknowledges to herself. Instead, it often manifests in her behaviour—in her daily choices to put her child's needs before her partner's and her own.

Early parenting and the sensual rival

Beyond birth comes nursing and physical relationship with an infant, and these are enmeshed with sexuality, with the ebb and flow of ovulation and menses, of sexual desire.

Adrienne Rich[33]

When I took my baby boy to the zoo for the first time, we saw zebras and giraffes and witnessed a tiger leap. We delighted in watching a family of gibbons. While the father swung about, the mother and baby gibbon grappled in a round of mock battles. When baby's attacks became too truculent, mother swiped him in a giant blow, sending him sliding across the floor, cartoon-like. Baby would then dive back to her, but instead of continuing the mêlée, he'd collapse into her chest and begin suckling.

It struck me that my baby and I spend our time together in similar ways—breastfeeding, wrestling, cuddling, biting and making silly sounds that could easily come from the wild. It also struck me that taking my son to the zoo for the first time may have been more exciting than any date I'd ever been on.

The intimacies of mother and child, whether ape or human, are so physically and emotionally deep that nothing else can compare.

Ayelet Waldman became notorious for publishing one thought: that she loved her husband more than her children.

So outraged were mother's groups across the US by her 2005 *New York Times* essay, 'Truly, Madly, Guiltily,'[34] that Waldman was called forth by Oprah to defend herself.

In the essay Waldman explored her transition from focusing on her partner to her child. She said, she found it perplexing when new mothers described sex as the last thing on their mind. Health care providers generally recommend waiting six weeks before resuming intercourse to allow time for the cervix to close and any tears or a repaired episiotomy to heal, but well past this time the women were blaming their lack of sex drive on exhaustion. Waldman didn't buy it; she felt something significant was missing from their explanations. Waldman wrote:

> . . . the real reason for this lack of sex, or at least the most profound, is that the wife's passion has been refocused. Instead of concentrating her ardor on her husband, she concentrates it on her babies. Where once her husband was the center of her passionate universe, there is now a new sun in whose orbit she revolves. Libido, as she once knew it, is gone, and in its place is all-consuming maternal desire.

Esther Perel, in *Mating in Captivity*,[35] argues that many of us fall in love with our children. Child-centrality, Perel argues, has reached unprecedented, almost cult-like heights. The sociologist Tina Miller even suggests that children are replacing the father as the head of the household.[36]

Discussing maternal desire at my mothers' group, a woman replied, 'With your child it's a different kind of love. It blows you away. I wasn't expecting that, the strength of it, and how wrapped up I am. It's hard to remember that you also love your husband. It sucks a lot of love out of you. I'm so preoccupied.'

One of the secrets of motherhood is that many women experience more intimacy with their children than with their partners. The touching, kissing, stroking and tending involved in the everyday care of young children can be sensual expressions of love.

If, as Perel contends, we fall in love with our babies as we once fell in love with lovers, we do so, similarly, to the exclusion of everybody else. As in any three-way relationship, someone soon feels left out. Within the context of a new family, it's usually dad: mummy has other things on her mind, and sex is rarely one of them.

Perel believes that the transition from two people to three is one of the most profound changes a couple experiences, and that it can take years to come to terms with its effects. We enter parenthood, she writes, with strong sexual identities. And then a child enters the love pair and everything shifts—how we see ourselves, our relationship to our friends, families and bodies, our priorities, our resources, our work life, and especially our ideas about freedom and responsibility. Becoming a family means less time, privacy, freedom, sleep . . . and sex drive.

The physical play and intimacy between mother and child is part of what Noelle Oxenhandler calls 'the eros of parenthood'. In her book of that title she writes, 'Non-orgasmic, but nevertheless intensely sensual forms of embodied connection are at the heart of loving parent–child attachment, and part of the spectrum of affectionate exchange between individuals generally.'[37] As Perel points out, this type of sensuality is more akin to female sexuality in general—diffuse and subjective rather than genital-focused.

Men can undergo a sexual shift alongside their partner's transition. Their sex drive may diminish during pregnancy, in the delivery room, or after the birth, as it's difficult for many men to see their former lover in this new entity, the mother. Yet most men don't openly discuss their lowered libido. Not only is it risky to diss the sex appeal of mothers in these politically correct times, men also confront—consciously or not—a deep and ancient idea: the Madonna/whore complex, in which women are seen as either mother figures or sexual ones, never both. Eroticising the mother of their child, Perel writes, feels 'too regressive, too incestuous, too oedipal'.[38] She advises men to healthily objectify their partner; anything to distinguish her from 'the mother'. Alternatively, a man's sex drive may not dimish at all. Instead, his unmet sexual needs may fester.

Sex post-baby rarely happens in a spontaneous flurry. It's not like you're out having a gorgeous dinner in a gorgeous dress, thinking about what you want to do to your lover when you get home. More likely you're having leftovers at home, thinking about what your partner hasn't done around the house.

The family bed

I was told that in Japan it is common for mothers to have one big futon where she and all her children sleep, while the father sleeps alone in another part of the house. Indeed, for thousands of years sleeping with children has been standard practice for women. In many countries it is still customary. Having a family bed ensures that the child is warm and suits small houses. It may also improve night-time breastfeeding and sleeping for young children. There is some evidence, however, that babies who sleep with their mothers nurse more frequently than babies who sleep solo.

Most Westerners haven't *deliberately* embraced the family bed, partly because there are conflicting beliefs about its safety. Nevertheless, many couples battling their children's sleep disturbances have resigned themselves to waking up and bringing their discontented darlings to mummy or daddy's bed. Although sleeping with infants is seen as a temporary solution to nighttime waking, it often becomes habitual.

The family bed often inadvertently demotes the adult relationship to second string. Having children in their bed limits the couple's sex life. While in theory they can have sex elsewhere, parents of young children rarely have the motivation. Loss of couple time can lead to resentment, feelings of neglect, and celibacy. For a single mother, bed-sharing can replace her need for physical intimacy. If children become used to sleeping against a parent's warm body, they may not want to return to their own room. So the family bed can lessen a couple's sensual bond over time.

Having experienced both the family bed with our first child and having my second baby sleep in a different room, I can attest that there are wonders to each arrangement. Sleeping with my daughter was sumptuous. I would hold her against my chest and breathe her in throughout the night. I felt closer to her than to my son, who was religiously tucked into a bassinette beside the bed and then, after a few months, transferred to a cot in his very own room.

And yet. The family bed was one of leakage, where vomit, baby urine, litres of breast milk, and tears fell. It was not a place of conversation or book reading or holding my husband. In fact, having my husband there, on the other side of my little girl gave me licence to devour her baby scent, hot-water-bottle body and velveteen cheeks and view him like a watercolor: abstract and safe.

A friend of mine has always slept with her two children. Her husband, after many years of enduring these cramped quarters, has taken to sleeping in his daughter's room . . . in her single bed . . . under a butterfly blanket. How incongruent: such an ultra-masculine man asleep beneath a plethora of butterflies. But this is another reality of parenthood. We stop loving our partners the way we used to. In focusing so singularly on the needs of our children, we unwittingly focus less on our partners.

Parenthood and marital satisfaction

Children do the strangest things to romance. In the 2004 movie *Before Sunset*, a character says, 'I feel like I'm running a small nursery with someone I used to date.' In a study of 93 married couples over a 10-year period, the psychologist Lawrence Kurdek identified two typical periods of relationship decline (defined as a decrease in marital passion, satisfaction, shared activities, and partner agreement).[39] Generally, things started off delightfully, declined fairly rapidly over the first four years, then stabilised . . . and then declined again in about the eighth year of marriage. Not long after from the notorious seven-year itch.

The first decline boiled down to 'normal adjustment to new roles'. The second was intertwined with the arrival of children. Kurdek also found that couples with children had lower marital quality after one year of marriage, and experienced steeper declines in marital quality, than couples without children. Other research has found that the wish to have a child increases happiness, but when the baby is born, happiness decreases, especially among fathers.[40]

In a 2003 analysis, Jean Twenge and Keith Campbell analysed 97 studies that compared the marital satisfaction of people with and without children, and correlated it with number of children. Unsurprisingly, mums reported loss of sleep and acute tiredness, a sense of jail-like confinement to the home, guilt at not being better mothers, worry about their appearance, and other dissatisfactions. Dads felt burdened by economic pressures resulting from their wife's withdrawal from the workplace, and reported general disenchantment with the parental role and a decline in their wife's sexual responsiveness.[41]

Numerous studies have shown that in modern Western society, conflicts over the sharing of housework, childcare and other responsibilities are common sources of friction. Women are often expected to take on a primarily caregiving role for the child, whereas men may be expected to take on a greater breadwinning role. A child can also threaten the parents' career track. All that social climbing for nil?

Twenge and Campbell found that parenthood is harder among younger birth cohorts and harder in more recent years. I wonder what it tells us that we increasingly can't cope and our marriages can't take the hard work of marriage. They note: 'For many people today, the preparenthood adult period is one of extraordinary freedom and self-focus. Consequently, there may be a greater contrast between young adult life and the early years of parenthood, a contrast that may make the transition more difficult and lead to greater marital dissatisfaction.'[42] For many of us, life BC (before children) centred around choosing pleasure, be it via cash, romance, a career, friendships, leisure, relaxing, or travelling. This gap is further accentuated when couples have children later in life, when they are accustomed to such pleasures and freedoms.

The implications of Twenge and Campbell's meta-analysis are rather depressing. They found that parents had significantly lower marital satisfaction than non-parents across 90 studies, and that there was a significant negative correlation between marital satisfaction and number of children. In fact, only 38 per cent of mothers of infants had high marital satisfaction, compared with 62 per cent of childless women, although the difference was less for women with older children. Parenthood had a stronger negative effect on women's marital satisfaction than on men's, and mothers of infants were the most dissatisfied. High socioeconomic groups also showed more marital dissatisfaction with parenthood than middle-class and low socioeconomic groups, leading the authors to write, 'Parenthood has a greater effect on marital satisfaction when one is particularly well educated or well-off.'[43] Amazing really, considering all those nanny hours.

A 2009 Swedish study explored changes in the relationships of 184 couples with small children. From the first interview to the second, four years later, couples reported a decrease in marital quality, especially with the birth of additional kids. Although the average frequency of sex hadn't changed since the first survey—once or twice a month—being too tired for it had become a bigger problem.[44]

But what good is it to know that a decrease in marital satisfaction after the birth of a child is often due to role conflicts and restriction of freedom? Perhaps we can use this fact as a guide to foster more equitable sharing of responsibilities; to prompt us to praise our partner for his love and his parenting efforts, thereby fostering feelings of closeness to the children and to the marriage,[45] and to use these findings to inform more reasonable expectations of love, partnership and child-raising. And perhaps, most importantly, we can use this information to stick up our finger at statistics and be one of the couples that make intimacy a priority, and keep our partnership sensuous.

Of course, strong, healthy marriages continue to function well after children enter the scene. Unstable relationships, on the other hand, can deteriorate. Children add much to a life, to the extent that they sometimes seem like the very meaning of it all. This meaningfulness grants many parents the grit to handle the reduction in satisfaction, adult sexuality and individual freedoms involved in parenting. However, neglecting the other person's sexual needs in a relationship is dangerous. As Catherine Kohler-Riessman notes,[46] for men sexuality is one of the main ways of achieving intimacy, and its absence often creates discontent, loneliness and emotional emptiness.

Rekindling maternal desire

With motherhood, much of what once gave you pleasure is zapped from your life. Things that you used to enjoy become quickly categorised as self-indulgent. Shopping for yourself is replaced by Costco trips, buying toilet paper by the barrel. Bikram yoga is replaced by baby ballet. And sex, goodness, is replaced by reading the same bedtime story night after night.

During courtship, libido has ample time to *unfold*. The slow build-up of sexual energy, heightened anticipation and spontaneity is what fuels desire. Family life, on the other hand, operates on routine and domesticity, which threaten the sensual process, as does maternal fatigue.

Many men have come a long way domestically and help us more than ever before. It wasn't all that long ago that we were supposed to greet our husband after work with a drink for him in one hand and his slippers in the other, while simpering, 'What else can I get for you, sweetie?' Yet we women are still ruled by The List—that all-consuming list of things to do, to buy, to finish. The List extends beyond the kitchen cupboard. It sinks into the laundry room. Creeps into the garden bed. Nestles into the children's toy chest. Frightens us in the bedroom mirror.

No space is free. There is always more to do, more to mend, and more not to forget. And, of course, there is always more to buy, fashioning us closer to the MILF, the 'mother I'd like to fuck'.

How are we to unwind when we are always winding? How are we to unfold when we are always—literally—folding? The endlessness of the list prevents many women from living sensually and being able to relax 'in the present'.

When we are constantly squeezed for time, former pastimes such as hobbies, exercise or sex can come to feel almost hedonistic. Unless we commit to keeping them a priority, such pleasures can fall right to the bottom of The List—below cleaning out the fridge and reheeling our shoes.

Worst of all, The List is invisible. Many of us grow resentful that our partners don't seem to see it, that The List is ours alone.

In a scene in *Sex in the City* just before Miranda and Steve break up, Carrie asks Miranda what's wrong. Miranda replies, 'I don't know. It's like he's a kid and I end up nagging him all the time. I'm Mean Mommy . . . and believe me, no one wants to fuck Mean Mommy.'

The List is a product of gender norms, whereby women serve the family's needs. But as satisfying as it can be to prepare a hot meal on a cold night and to nurture our loved ones, what is the cost of not nurturing ourselves?

A balance is called for, a balance between serving ourselves and serving our family. Even though on many days, if not most, this seems impossible.

With motherhood, libido often gets pushed into the drawer along with paracetamol and recipes we may one day try. Setting our love life aside is not often a conscious decision. Rather, it is the result of many small, subtle decisions: each time we turn away from our partner's embrace. Each choice not to engage with our own sensuality. Instead, we wait for the right moment: when we feel rested, when we feel sexy, when there is free time . . . But empty spaces in a mother's life are few and far between. And when they do blissfully appear they often get filled with a sigh, a cup of tea, and feet up for the first time in hours. Not a penis.

Although we may convince ourselves that our sensuality is no longer so important, for many of us, seeing ourselves as sexual beings is fundamental to our emotional and physical health. It's also what can keep relationships dynamic, providing that elusive spark.

There are, however, ways to create space in a hectic life so that sensuality is within reach. To begin, awareness of the sexual stalemate, and a decision to do something about it, is crucial. Then evaulate how you divide your time throughout the week, and work to redirect some of your creative sensuality. Take heed of sexologist's common suggestion: quickies or planned sex. For parents, waiting until the mood strikes is the equivalent of a teenage girl waiting to be discovered by a modelling agent in a suburban mall.

Instead of seizing the perfect moment, be ready for any moment. When the toddler goes down for an afternoon kip, grab your partner and make your way to the bedroom for some sensual time out.

Scheduling sex may seem unerotic, but it at least means sex can take place. If not consciously made room for, desire may visit less often than the Tooth Fairy. After all, much of our previous dating experience contained an element of scheduling: booking a time and place, bathing and beautifying. Yet, because we did these things in the context of seduction, of dating, it is immune to criticism whereas in the context of the domestic or marital, planned intimacy seems forced. It's a fairytale that everything lusty has to come about spontaneously. Consciously creating space for the sensual to *unfold* is a way to keep eros in sight.

As we will see in Chapter 5, desire encompasses the effort we make. Greater effort indicates greater desire, and rewarding behaviour is self-reinforcing.

Given that anticipation is one of the greatest igniters of desire, it makes sense to play with this. Although we can't pretend to be swept off our feet, we can still enjoy the lead-up to sex. Erotic tension can be achieved by knowing adults-only time is scheduled and has been given priority. Merely being alone together *sans* children and doing things you both like can reaffirm connection.

Plan sex the same way you plan a night out. As in: meet you in our bedroom on 30 October, nude.

Who knows what deliciousness might unfold?

5

Sex models: the mystery of female desire

After centuries of conditioning the female into the condition of perpetual girlishness called femininity, we cannot remember what femaleness is. Though feminists have been arguing for years that there is a self-defining female energy, and a female libido that is not expressed merely in response to demands by the male, and a female way of being and experiencing the world, we are still not close to understanding what it might be.

Germaine Greer[1]

Figuring out how men and women experience desire, arousal and sexual satisfaction has given science a real task to chew on. Indeed, after all the theories, lab experiments, case studies, ethnographies, postal surveys, vaginal photo-plethysmographs, psychoanalysis, brain scanning, measuring of hormone levels and pretty much everything else you could think of, we still don't really know what makes men and women tick. And we certainly know less about the latter. Until recently, medical science has paid little attention to female sexuality, but now, with the race to procure a pink Viagra, our sexual happiness is suddenly at the forefront of the 'big pharma' (pharmaceutical) agenda.

One of the biggest problems standing in the way of understanding our inherent sexual nature is that culture, religion, social norms, the media and the theories currently fashionable in academia all have a knack of biasing the whole shebang. Also, throughout history, it has rarely been safe for a woman to have surplus, free-flowing, unrestrained libido. Because of this we don't know how female sexuality manifests in its free form. To nail down what female sexuality is—its true scope and essence—we need to observe it free-range, outside the parameters of our patriarchal society.

Given that our own biographies, our past and current romantic entanglements and our particular brain chemistry influence our sexuality, much of what constitutes sexual desire is subjective or individually unique. Yet our sexual identity exists in the context of a shared culture, in which religion, media and gender norms play a pivotal role.

This chapter explores the psychology of libido, and then outlines the different models scientists have come up with to map our sexual response. Each model emphasises different aspects of physiology, psychology, relationships and cultural influences; getting the 'right' model is crucial, as it is used as *the* criterion to determine what is sexually 'normal' versus 'sexually dysfunctional'. Finally, we'll look at the role of culture and gender in shaping our collective desires.

Eros, from Freud to *jouissance*
Eros

The term eros comes from Greek mythology. Eros was the god of love, and was worshipped as a fertility deity. He was most often depicted as a young winged boy with a bow and arrows—either golden with dove feathers, to incite love, or leaden with owl feathers, to cause indifference. His Roman counterpart, Cupid, has appeared on Valentine's Day cards forever. Traditionally, Eros was the patron of male love, while Aphrodite ruled the love between men and women. Eros is now a common term for sexual desire. Throughout the book I use it to invoke sensuality and fleshy desire. I also use it interchangeably with libido or sex drive.

In Latin, *libido* referred to desire and lust, but it was Freud's use of the term in 1909 that led to its mainstream popularity. Indeed, before relatively recent advances in medical science—vaginal photoplethysmographs and brain activity scans—one's libido was likely to be examined while reclining on a leather couch.

Sigmund Freud, Carl Jung, Alfred Adler, Jacques Lacan and other leaders of psychoanalytic thought have had much to say on the nature of human libido.

Freud's libido

Freud believed we enter the world as unbridled pleasure-seekers. Beyond the basic animal instincts to seek food and avoid pain, our motivation is organised and directed by two instincts or drives: sexuality (*Eros*) and the death drive (*Thanatos*).

Freud thought that both of these instincts were powered by a form of internal psychic and sexual energy that he called the libido. He argued that libido is the single most important motivating force in adult life.[2] Although libido encompasses sexuality, it embraces the 'energy of all the life instincts'.[3]

For Freud, sexual drive was characterised by a gradual build-up to a peak in intensity, followed by a sudden decrease of excitement, it worked like the urges behind eating, drinking, urinating and defecating, all of which were sexual or libidinous.[4] Freud gave sexual drives centrality in human life and human behaviour and redefined the term 'sexuality' to envelop any form of pleasure derived from the body.

Freud believed Eros needed to be civilised, channelled and controlled lest libido run free. Were it to do so, mayhem would rule, with incest, rape, murder. To Freud, healthy individuals suppressed their libido so that they still got pleasure but avoided chaos.

Freudian libido develops in several distinct stages. Each stage brings frustrations, and if these are not successfully resolved, the libido may become dammed up, producing pathological traits in adulthood. 'Fixation' refers to a failure to progress to later stages of psychosexual development and can result from excessive frustration or excessive gratification of sexual urges. The goal of Freudian psychoanalysis is to bring the fixations of an immature individual to conscious awareness so that libidinal energy is freed up and available for conscious use.

Freud's first stage in the development of libido is the *oral stage*, which lasts from birth to about one year of age. At this time sexual drive or libido is focused in the mouth, primarily manifesting in sucking. The individual may be frustrated by having to wait on or be dependent on another person. Being fixated at this stage may lead to excessive oral stimulation later in life, such as by smoking, drinking or overeating.

In the *anal stage,* which occurs from about one to three years of age, the focus of erotic pleasure moves to defecating. Punitive training (or excessive reward) can lead to fixation at this stage, resulting in adult stinginess, stubbornness, withholding, pedantic cleanliness or messiness.

The *oedipal or phallic stage* occurs at around three to six years of age, when libidinal focus shifts to the sex organs. Critical episodes for development occur during this stage, and both boys and girls experience the 'Oedipus conflict': sexual desires for the mother/father. The child sees her father/mother as rivals for its affections. A boy may fear that his father knows about his longing for his mother and will punish him for it. This fear is known as 'castration anxiety'. Children need to overcome their desire for the opposite-sex parent and identify with the same-sex parent.

Once the Oedipus conflict has been resolved, the child enters the *latency stage*, which lasts from about the age of six until 12. This is a period of rest during which no libido-related developmental events occur.

Finally, the *genital stage* occurs from puberty onwards, from about age 12 to 18. Pleasure, once again, is derived from the genitals. Feelings for the opposite sex are a source of anxiety—they act as reminders of the feelings once focused on the parents and the resulting trauma.[5]

According to Freud, the development of the human psyche involves three components: the id, the ego and the superego. Put simply, the id is the *biological* component, the ego is the *psychological* component, and the superego is the internalised *social* component.[6]

The *id* (literally the 'it') is the source of our libido, and the only structure present at birth. The id is the seat of basic drives and impulses, and operates primarily in visual and irrational terms. It lives in the immediate present and is unable to defer pleasure. After birth, part of the id differentiates into the *ego*, whose function is to translate the id's internal dream-like wishes into contact with actual objects. The ego provides an executive function, able to direct our libidinous desires in socially acceptable and achievable ways. The *superego* is the sum of our internalised social norms. The ideal adult state is characterised by a strong ego, a healthy superego and the ability to delay gratification.

According to Freud, when we are awake these three components are separated, but during sleep and fantasy the boundaries weaken and there is an 'open expression of otherwise controlled libidinous desires'. Awareness of these desires can result in sexual guilt or shame, yet repressing libidinal impulses can also negatively affect an individual's psychological wellbeing.[7]

Many of Freud's theories have been criticised as bourgeois and patriarchial, yet as the feminist Juliet Mitchell asserts, his theories are not a recommendation of a patriarchal society but an *analysis* of one.[8] Further, more recent researchers have found evidence that Freud's drives really do exist and have their roots in the limbic system, a primitive part of the brain that operates mostly below the horizon of consciousness.[9]

Since Freud, subsequent schools of psychoanalysis and psychology have broadened and reshaped the concept of libido to incorporate other non-sexual drives and emotions. Carl Jung was arguably the first to break away from Freud's it's-all-about-sex motif.

Jung and Adler: Freud's most important groupies

Carl Gustav Jung, a Swiss psychiatrist, was good mates with Sigmund Freud. They hung out a lot and collaborated intensively over six years during a pivotal time in the history of psychoanalysis.[10] For reasons unknown, in 1913 they broke off their friendship and never spoke again.

Jung found great success in his own theory, which he named 'analytical psychology', and which is recognised now as Jungian psychology. Jung, like Freud, believed that the unconscious determines personality. However, unlike Freud, he believed there are two layers to the unconscious:

- The *personal* unconscious (the unconscious of Freud's theory)—consisting of thoughts, memories and desires that are repressed or forgotten.
- The *collective* unconscious—a shared human spiritual heritage, a storehouse of latent memories inherited from our ancestral past.[11]

While Freud saw libido mostly through a sexual lens, Jung used the term to encompass the life force in all species: all creative energies, including hunger, thirst, sleep and will to survive. For Jung, although libido could have a sexual expression, it could also manifest in musical composition, for example.[12] Later theories of motivation have substituted the term 'drive' for libido.

Alfred Adler, an Austrian medical doctor and psychologist, was among the co-founders of the psychoanalytic movement. Adler was the first major figure to form an independent school of psychotherapy and personality theory. Adler would come to have an enormous effect on the disciplines of counselling and psychotherapy. He believed that the most basic human drive is the striving from 'inferiority' toward self-actualisation. He focused on the life experience of individuals rather than the sexually obsessed abstractions of Freud and the mysticism of Jung.[13]

Lacan and *jouissance*

The French come up with lots of cool ideas. *Jouissance* is one of them. According to the anthropologist Aleksandar Bošković, *jouissance* is untranslatable into English, but implies a state similar to bliss or enjoyment; the closest translation would be the feeling that comes with and follows after orgasm.[14] *Jouissance* also implies happiness connected with the possession of some valuable thing. It comes from the verb *jouir*, one of whose main meanings is 'to come'. Currently in France it is used almost exclusively in the sexual context.

French psychoanalyst and psychiatrist Jacques Lacan believed that there is a limit to pleasure which, if transgressed, becomes pain. The pleasure and pain of *jouissance* stem from early-childhood separation from the mother and the associated psychological creation of a symbolic object-cause-of-desire, which Lacan defined as 'object a'. The gap between us and the object can never be closed, we cannot reunify with the mother, so we are wired to perpetually chase that which we can never attain. A constant quest, the fantasy of unity, drives us and creates *jouissance*.

Lacan believed all desire springs from lack, and anxiety appears when this lack is in itself lacking. We desire and seek partners to fill the lack, but they will always fall short. Paradoxically, anxiety is also created if we get too close. We enjoy our lack and also fear the *jouissance* of the other. Desire involves attraction and repulsion, pleasure and pain, ecstasy and suffering. These opposing forces coexist within us, affecting our relationships at a subterranean level.

The Lacanian view of the sexuality of men sheds light on their tendency to objectify women. At a subconscious level, men see women as a proxy for the ultimate object they perpetually seek, yet they also fear engulfment by women. This leads to a proclivity to split their love objects, partitioning love from lust and positioning women as either 'virgin' or 'whore'. This can cause men to find themselves in desexualised, platonic love for the one and carnal lust for the other, but not both in a single woman.[15] This concept may illuminate the challenge of the transition from couple to family (Chapter 4), especially for the male who may be psychologically wired to chase . . . or run away.

Feminine *jouissance*

The French psychoanalyst Marie-Christine Laznik explains that Lacan 'introduced a jouissance outside the phallic order, a mystic jouissance, which he defined as a nonphallic, feminine jouissance'. This mystical *jouissance* is 'outside sex', but to attain it women must abandon trying to be their partner's 'object a'.[16] The feminist Luce Irigaray also believes women experience their *jouissance* in many more ways than men.[17] To overcome the obstacles culture puts before us, she argues, women should explore the *plurality* of our sexuality. We need to find ways to bring our real self to being, to establish our own values outside the limited definition of the objectifying gaze. We can define our own sexuality as we see fit. We don't need to fit neatly into society's definitions of what we should be.

Love, sex and the brain

In *A Midsummer Night's Dream*, Shakespeare gives the mischievous Puck a magical juice from a flower called 'love-in-idleness'. This juice, when applied to a sleeping person's eyelids, makes the victim fall in love with the first living thing he sees upon awakening, donkey or otherwise. Although not as fanciful, recent neurological research has shown that the choices we make when selecting bedfellows are in many ways out of our hands. Rather, they take place inside our brains.

Over the last decade the American anthropologist Helen Fisher has been looking at love, literally. With her research team, Fisher took brain scans of people in love and followed the circuitry of romance.[18] Subjects were shown two photographs, one neutral, the other of their loved one. When subjects looked at their beloved—*bang!*—parts of the brain linked to reward and pleasure became stimulated.

Love apparently activates the caudate nucleus, which houses a dense cluster of receptors for a neurotransmitter called . . . dopamine.

Dopamine, our own love potion, rivals Shakespeare's.

One of Fisher's central ideas is that romantic love is a universal human drive, stronger than the sex drive, thirst and hunger and sometimes even stronger than the will to live. She proposes that humans have three primary motivational circuits—*lust*, *attraction* and *attachment*—and that these brain systems have evolved to direct our mating and reproductive behaviour.

According to Fisher, each phase of falling in love activates different chemicals in the body. Stage one, lust, involves androgens and influences our libido. Driven by testosterone in both men and women, it's what causes us to seek sex (and is easily observed at closing time in bars across the country).

Stage two, attraction, starts when we spy an attractive potential mate. A powerful chain reaction is triggered by phenylethylamine, a natural amphetamine that increases physical and emotional energy and speeds information transfer between nerve cells, which in turn assists the release of dopamine, the pleasure chemical. AKA 'butterflies'. The combination of dopamine and norepinephrine makes us euphoric, bold and willing to take risks.

The third stage of love, attachment, involves oxytocin. Known as the 'commitment molecule', oxytocin is released upon orgasm, when a mother nurses her baby, and when long-time couples canoodle.

Much of our understanding about bonding comes from research with prairie voles, animals with high levels of oxytocin that mate for life. When scientists block oxytocin receptors in the rodents, they get randy and ditch their soul mates. And when the natural release of oxytocin is blocked in sheep and rats, they reject their own young. If you inject oxytocin into virgin female rats, on the other hand, it causes them to fawn over other females' young, nuzzling the pups and protecting them as if they were their own.

However, as the psychologist Brenda Schaeffer writes, 'While these brain circuits and emotions work with each other in a safe and fulfilling love relationship, they can and do function independently of one another. You can be bonded with one person, infatuated with another and have sex with yet a third person.'[19]

Romantic love is the result of what Fisher rather hilariously refers to as 'abnormalities' of dopamine, norepinephrine and another mood-altering chemical, serotonin. Exploring the similarities between love and obsessive–compulsive disorder (OCD), Italian psychiatrist Donatella Marazziti and her colleagues measured blood serotonin levels in 24 subjects who had fallen in love within the past six months and who obsessed about their love object for at least four hours every day . . . and discovered that their low serotonin levels matched those of OCD patients.[20] It suddenly makes sense . . . all those feckless things I've done, including once climbing uninvited through the bedroom window of a man with whom I was infatuated. 'Surprise!'

Unfortunately, according to Michael Liebowitz, the author of *The Chemicals of Love*, we develop a chemical *tolerance* to the person we're in a relationship with.[21] Over time, the individual who was initially responsible for igniting all those hormonal reactions in us becomes less of a turn-on. Our kisses become less lingering. Our sensuality transfers to other areas of our life, such as reselling items previously bought on eBay. Liebowitz believes the neuropharmacological basis of love lasts only for two to three years.

When it comes to sex, the brain interprets stimulation—*he looks delicious*—and then starts 'activating' other body parts (increased breathing rate, wet vagina, etc). In brain–sex research a lot of attention has been paid to the mechanisms of excitation and inhibition. Various chemicals in the body have been found to have remarkable effects—turning us on and off. The production of these chemicals is complex and affected by various parts of the brain.

Sexual inhibition

From the nervous system's perspective, inhibition appears to be more powerful than excitation. The Canadian psychologist James Pfaus says sexual inhibition is probably an adaptive response to keep individuals out of trouble, helping them avoid risky, inappropriate sexual behaviour. However, too much inhibition can lead to sexual dysfunction, including inhibited arousal, desire and/or diminished capacity to achieve sexual gratification.[22]

When we reach sexual satiety, inhibitory neural systems are activated and serotonin is released, which is why orgasm can provide a rush of euphoria, followed by a prolonged period of relaxation. Other inhibitory chemicals include the morphine-like opioids—including endorphins—which are released in the brain during orgasm and give us the sensation of satisfaction. As we have seen in Chapter 4, prolactin, secreted by the pituitary gland to stimulate lactation, is another substance that turns us off sex.

Studying sexual inhibition is critical if we are to understand how certain events or 'prosexual' drugs—such as booze, cocaine and sexual pharmaceuticals—result in a loss of sexual inhibition.[23]

Sexual excitation

When we encounter something that 'does it' for us, the endocrine system is activated, hormones are secreted, and changes occur in our bodies. Attention and desire are stimulated by the activation of the neurotransmitter dopamine and hormones called melanocortins. Sexual arousal is stimulated by the activation of neurotransmitters including noradrenaline and oxytocin.

Dopamine, norepinephrine, melanocortin and oxytocin act in the hypothalamic and limbic regions of the brain to stimulate sexual arousal. Dopamine is associated with the brain's pleasure and reward system. Dopamine agonists (agents that activate dopamine receptors) have been found to stimulate sexual arousal and excitement in both rats and humans. Norepinephrine is also a stimulator of sexual desire and is involved in arousal, attention and mood.[24]

Desire and the ovulatory cycle

Female sexual desire, genital arousal and emotional response to sexual stimuli change across the ovulatory cycle. Some research has shown that women initiate and solicit sexual activity around the time they ovulate.[25] A number of women report that their libido rises steadily a week prior to ovulation, peaks around the time of ovulation, then declines over the next week.[26] Increases in subjective arousal and desire while watching porn—a common scientific aid in measuring libido—are also reported to be greater during the follicular (ovulation) phase than the luteal phase (the stage of the menstrual cycle after ovulation).[27]

A 2007 American study found that the ovulatory cycle affected the tip earnings of lap dancers. The dancers earned $335 during oestrus (when women are most fertile), $260 during the luteal phase, and only $185 when they were menstruating. Those who were on the Pill had no such peak during oestrus.[28]

Desire and arousal

In a 2003 article titled 'What can animal models tell us about human response?'[29], James Pfaus noted that animal sexual behavior is in many ways comparable to our own and controlled by similar/identical neurochemical and hormonal systems. Like us, animals experience sexual arousal, desire, reward and inhibition. Female rats prefer to control the initiation and rate of sexual contact, and male rats are excited by females that require some form of courtship and will work hard to get even small rewards. Pfaus believes that in *all* mammalian species, sexual behavior appears to have similar processes and endpoints.[30]

Sexual *arousal* in humans and other animals can be defined as increased automatic activation that prepares the body for sexual activity. *Desire*, on the other hand, is harder to pinpoint. The Diagnostic and Statistical Manual of Mental Disorders (DSM) categorises arousal disorders as independent from desire disorders, arousal being generally marked by blood flow to genitals and erectile tissues versus a 'psychological' sexual interest. But desire may be shaped by the presence of responses that define arousal, and there are those who believe desire and arousal are one and the same, or so interlaced that they are impossible to separate.[31]

The most prevalent view is that desire refers to a baseline interest in sex, or to our sexual appetite, which can be activated by endogenous and/or exogenous stimuli, while arousal refers to physical and mental feelings of sexual excitement and awareness of genital sensations.[32] Desire can be experienced before, during, or after arousal. For Pfaus, our sex drive is largely defined by our moment-to-moment sexual arousability, our ability to respond to hormonal and neurochemical changes that signal desire and arousal. But this is just a ticket to the gig. The remainder, he says, demands a mix of instinct, learning, feedback, looking for mates, figuring out who is receptive, and then courting them.[33]

The concept of desire, Pfaus believes, should also encompass *effort*. Much of this takes place before sexual interaction, for example 'bar pressing in rats or flower giving in people'.[34] Ha! Furthermore, these actions can be considered 'sexual' if they occur in anticipation of a sexual reward, such as when we buy a dress with the sole purpose of having it unzipped.

Neural mechanisms exist that allow stimulation received during sexual contact to be perceived as rewarding. So in addition to making us feel amorous, desire encompasses the work people/rats will perform to obtain sexual rewards and the excitement displayed in anticipation of such rewards.

And, as any dog owner knows, reward alters subsequent behavior. Thus for Pfaus desire is participatory, with greater effort indicating greater desire.[35]

Males can be a bit slow to respond, as Pfaus observes:

During copulation, female rats control the initiation and pacing of copulation by soliciting mounts from males. A female makes a headwise orientation to the male and then runs away, forcing the male to chase her. If the male is sluggish or nonresponsive, the female may increase the strength of her solicitations, to the point of kicking the male in the head before the runaway or even mounting the male if he does not respond to previous enticements.[36]

Usually, however, boys will do anything to get their girl. Pfaus writes:

In male rats, these behaviors have included performance in obstruction boxes, straight-alley running, maze learning, crossing of electrified grids, nose pokes and other attempts to 'get to' a potential sex partner . . . Indeed, to gain access to receptive females, male guinea pigs will learn to run an alley, male pigeons will learn to peck keys, and male stickleback fish will learn to swim through rings.[37]

And how many human males won't even buy us a drink?

Blondes versus brunettes

If you believe the power of reward is secondary to innate attraction, get this. According to research, rats show a sexual preference for specific features. Rather than being driven by instinct to maximise reproductive fitness, many such preferences are learned through association with sexual reward.

Exploring the conditioned preferences in the seasonally monogamous Japanese quail, Susan Nash and Michael Domjan allowed male quails to copulate with females of different plumage color, either brown or blonde. They chose to spend more time near females whose color was the same as that of females they had copulated with previously.[38] So, although the study does little to settle the brunettes-versus-blondes debate, it suggests that sexual conditioning is a more powerful force than many imagine.

Hurts so good

Many scientists believe that low libido is caused by changes in the brain chemicals that regulate sexual desire. Chronic low libido, for example, may result from an imbalance in the inhibitory and excitatory neurotransmitter system and hormones.

Discussing this, Pfaus writes that central excitation and inhibition both activate the autonomic nervous system. Life-threatening stimuli activate the sympathetic arm of the system, increasing blood and oxygen supply to muscles and organs that need them, and turning off blood flow to the genitals. However, in response to sexual stimuli, both arms of the autonomic nervous system are activated, with the sympathetic system increasing blood flow from the heart and the parasympathetic system increasing blood flow to the genitals. In other words, a small degree of threat or stress in humans, something naughty (infidelity, outdoor sex) or mildly painful (hot wax, spanking), can be arousing.

Translated into a sexual situation, such arousal could be directed to sexual activity, and repetition can make it a necessary antecedent to it.[39]

The arousing nature of pain has been studied with the help of our rat friends. Although punishment and shock can suppress a variety of appetitive and consummatory behaviors in rats, a number of studies show that short-term pain (tail pinch) stimulates mounting in sexually sluggish or inactive male rats, and reduces the number of intromissions required for ejaculation in sexually active males. Indeed both male and female rats will readily cross electrified grids to gain access to sexually receptive partners.[40]

After male rats learned to suppress their copulatory advances toward sexually non-receptive females, researchers gave them low to moderate doses of alcohol. Tequila perhaps? This resulted in an increased proportion of males attempting to mount non-receptive females. As well, many males ejaculated despite never gaining vaginal penetration (I'm not even going to go there). So, for rats at least, low to moderate doses of alcohol can release sexual behavior from inhibition.[41] However if they are too boozed up, as human males can attest, sex is the last thing on their minds.

Because sexual behavior in rats can be altered by pharmaceutical agents, Pfaus has received consulting grants and been on the advisory boards of a number of pharmaceutical companies. To treat chronic low libido, Pfaus sees future drug therapies targeting the excitatory and/or inhibitory functions of the central nervous system, the aim being to tone down the inhibitory function and/or boost dopamine and noradrenaline levels.[42] More on this in Chapter 9.

Sex models: from the swinging '60s to the present

Although the neuroscientist's view of libido is fascinating, there is more to it than physiology. In this section we'll look at some important models of human sexual behavior, from Masters and Johnson's to more recent ones, to expand our understanding from the purely physiological to the psychological, relational and (to a degree) cultural.

To place these models in a wider context, the diagram outlines the broad dimensions of libido and human sexual response and gives examples of each.

Formulating a precise model of sexual human behaviour is so important, and so fiercely debated, because what is defined as 'normal' affects what is defined as 'dysfunctional', and what is defined as dysfunctional affects the marketing of pharmaceuticals to alter our sexual response. The defining of 'normal' versus 'abnormal' sexuality also directly affects psychology, sex therapy, health care, science and medicine.

The evolution of sex models brings to light the complexities of understanding libido, desire, arousal, and how men and women experience these areas differently.

The Masters and Johnson model

The work of William Masters and Virginia Johnson has had a rock-star impact on our understanding of human sexuality. They described sexual response as primarily the result of increased blood flow to various parts of the body, called *vasocongestion,* and increased muscle tension, called *myotonia.* In 1966, Masters and Johnson presented a four-stage physiological model of sexual response: excitement, plateau, orgasm and resolution.[43]

The first stage, excitement, occurs as a result of erotic physical or mental stimulation. Both sexes experience an increase in heart and breathing rate, muscle tension, and blood flow to the genitals and other erogenous zones, resulting in swelling, lubrication and erection.

Next, the plateau phase is a period of enhanced sexual excitement prior to orgasm. It usually lasts a number of minutes, but if prolonged may yield more intense orgasms. The man's penis becomes fully erect and he may start secreting seminal or pre-ejaculatory fluid. For many women reaching this stage is often enough to satisfy them, but for others, staying on the plateau leads to fury.

Orgasm, or climax, is the shortest of all the phases, usually measured in seconds. At orgasm, all physiological responses peak. In women, orgasm produces muscular contractions and intense sensations. Orgasms may also play a role in fertilisation: the muscular spasms may aid the locomotion of sperm up the vaginal walls into the uterus.

In the resolution phase, the body eases back to its pre-excited state. Men experience a refractory (recovery) period in which orgasm is temporarily out of the picture. For women, however, further stimulation may cause a return to the plateau stage, allowing for multiple orgasms. However, most women, despite a biological advantage, have never had the pleasure of experiencing this. *La petite mort*, the little death, as the French describe orgasm, is elusive to many. The sexologist Alfred Kinsey reported in the 1950s that only 14 per cent of women were multi-orgasmic; by 1970, the proportion was 16 per cent. Today, it's reported as 15 to 25 per cent.[44] Master and Johnson categorised

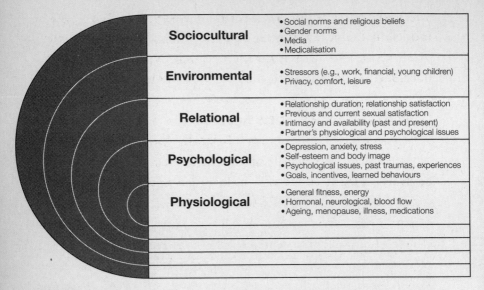

Sociocultural	• Social norms and religious beliefs • Gender norms • Media • Medicalisation
Environmental	• Stressors (e.g., work, financial, young children) • Privacy, comfort, leisure
Relational	• Relationship duration; relationship satisfaction • Previous and current sexual satisfaction • Intimacy and availability (past and present) • Partner's physiological and psychological issues
Psychological	• Depression, anxiety, stress • Self-esteem and body image • Psychological issues, past traumas, experiences • Goals, incentives, learned behaviours
Physiological	• General fitness, energy • Hormonal, neurological, blood flow • Ageing, menopause, illness, medications

Figure 1: Libido and human sexual response, Bella Ellwood-Clayton 2012

sexual complaints according to which stage of the four was affected. They defined women as having 'primary orgasmic dysfunction' and 'situational orgasmic dysfunction', a step up from the pre-1970s label of frigidity.[45]

Despite its accuracy in describing the physicality of sexual arousal, the Masters and Johnson sex model was criticised for ignoring desire and the emotional aspects of sexuality. By focusing on orgasm as the climax of a sexual encounter, their model also de-emphasised other forms of sexual pleasure. Nor did it allow for individual or gender variation, suggesting that most people proceed smoothly through discrete stages when for many women this is not the case.

Nevertheless, during the 1970s and 1980s, while hair went from bad to big, the Masters and Johnson model was expanded upon by several researchers. These new models included emotional aspects of sexual response and often recognised that a peak emotional experience doesn't necessarily coincide with a peak physiological one.

Other models of sexual response

Whereas Masters and Johnson's model focused mainly on physiological changes, the sex therapist Helen Singer Kaplan came up with a condensed model, the triphasic model of sexual response, which included the ever-important 'desire' factor:

- desire—it all starts with desire: a psychological interest in sex before any physical changes occur
- excitement—physiological arousal and which may or may not lead to orgasm
- resolution—a return to the pre-aroused state; cigarette optional.[46]

Kaplan observed that sexual problems fell into categories and that it was possible to be inhibited in one area and still function normally in the other two. A woman with low desire, for example, might not initate sex, but could become aroused and have orgasms if induced into sexual activity. Kaplan's therapeutic experience also led her to believe that sexual desire problems were the hardest to remedy.

Psychiatrist and sex therapist Harold Lief also proposed that desire was a distinct phase in the model of sexual response. He suggested that women who chronically failed to respond to sexual initiation should be diagnosed with 'inhibited sexual desire'.[47]

The sex therapists Bernie Zilbergeld and Carol Ellison massaged Masters and Johnson's and Kaplan's models together into a five-stage model, beginning again with desire or interest and ending with satisfaction.[48] Whalen and Roth proposed a cognitive model of sexuality, adding a 'perception' element before sexual arousal to reflect that we first must *interpret* stimuli as arousing.[49] They also emphasised the evaluation process in the lead-up to and during sex: *How do I look? What's going wrong? What does this mean?*, which can potentially interfere with sexual response.

In the late 1980s, John Bancroft incorporated motivational factors and arousability within his model's first phase: appetite or drive. This was followed by three more phases—central arousal, genital response and peripheral arousal. Bancroft's second phase, central arousal, refers to the excitation of the central nervous system.[50]

Further pushing sex models into the psychosocial realm, in the late 1990s David Reed proposed the ESP model of sexual response. Leaving the paranormal aside, his erotic stimulus pathway had four stages: seduction, sensation, surrender, reflection.[51]

Seduction entails all those things we might do to entice someone, and ourselves, into sexual liaisons: dressing well, wearing cologne or perfume, making eye contact, sending erotic texts or emails, buying sweet inconsequential gifts, manufacturing 'the right time' or 'right place' or soliciting sex. These processes often involve memories and rituals.

Sensations such as sight, sound, taste, smell and touch, as well as imagination and fantasy, all have the potential to arouse. Potential is dependent on how we interpret sensations, which is often based on prior learning and cultural surroundings.

Orgasm, according to Reed, is all about power. Experiencing orgasm requires surrendering control, and can require trust in ourselves and our partner. Also important is ridding ourselves of anxiety about how we look, how we sound, and how we judge our sexual performance. The letting-go process is an essential element of a sensual life and one that a pill cannot neatly remedy.

In the fourth stage, reflection, we look back over our sexual experience and examine how we felt about it. If we enjoyed it, many of us look forward to the next cycle, beginning with seduction. If it was a negative experience, we may avoid future sexual encounters. Song choice: 'Hit the road, Jack'.

In keeping with the late '90s attitude, Beverly Whipple and Karen Brash-McGreer wanted their model to have a bit of everything. They took Masters and Johnson's four phases—excitement, plateau, orgasm and resolution—added desire at the beginning *à la* Kaplan, and then laid Reed's circular seduction, sensation, surrender and reflection over the top, creating a diagram that would make management consultants weep.[52]

In 2005, Michael Perelman presented the sexual tipping-point model, which illustrates the multidimensional nature of a variety of sexual dysfunctions in both men and women. The big point here is that there's a *threshold* between sexual inhibition and excitation, which can be inhibited or facilitated by a mixture of both psychosocial and physiological factors. It's the interplay between excitation and inhibition that determines an individual's level of sexual responsiveness at any given time. Sexual tipping points are thought to exist throughout the phases of the sexual response cycle.[53]

Now there are, of course, many non-sexual reasons why women have sex. Cindy Meston and David Buss explored women's varying combinations of motivations for sex and found that they included:

- pleasure—sexual gratification, orgasm
- love—emotional and spiritual connection
- the thrill of conquest—competing for a mate, stealing another person's partner, revenge
- green-eyed desire—mate guarding, provoking jealousy, trading up
- duty—to nurture, to do what is expected
- adventure—curiosity, variety, mate evaluation
- ego boost—to feel attractive/boost self-esteem, to regain dignity
- barter and trade—to obtain resources (money, house, clothes), social status.[54]

Rosemary Basson's sexual response model
Rosemary Basson has published some 50 peer-reviewed articles, many of them concentrating on reconceptualising the female sexual response. She has also facilitated the attempt

by an international consensus committee to revise definitions of women's sexual dysfunctions. And Basson, like many of the key researchers studying sexual function and dysfunction, has ties to pharmaceutical companies; she was a consultant for Pfizer and Solvay. Pfizer is the largest pharmaceutical company in the world. The same pharmaceutical company that, in 2009, pleaded guilty to the largest health care fraud in US history and received the largest criminal penalty ever levied for illegal marketing of four of its drugs. As this was Pfizer's fourth such settlement with the US Department of Justice in the previous ten years, they were given a title shared by Charlie Sheen: repeat offender.

Basson's model of female sexual response is what she calls an 'intimacy-based sex response cycle'. It starts with intimacy needs, which cause women to seek out and be receptive to sexual stimuli; then biological and psychological factors affect the processing of these stimuli; then sexual arousal kicks in, followed by sexual desire. This creates more arousal and pleasure and a positive outcome emotionally and physically, culminating in the ultimate goal—enhanced intimacy.

So the model is seemingly *all* about intimacy. Sexual stimuli, arousal and desire are tools to achieve intimacy. Basson thus defines women as intimacy hunters.

According to Basson, men and women have different sexual response systems, different sexual motivations, and women are *ultimately manipulative*. Like Meston and Buss, Basson believes women have many reasons for engaging in sexual activity other than sexual hunger or drive, as the traditional sex models suggest. She thinks a number of mostly non-sexual 'rewards' or 'gains' motivate women to have sex:

> When a woman senses a potential opportunity to be sexual with her partner, although she may not 'need' to experience arousal and resolution for her own sexual well-being, she is nevertheless motivated to deliberately do whatever is necessary to facilitate a sexual interaction as she expects potential benefits that, though not strictly sexual, are very important.[55]

In other words, women use sex to get what they want . . . which is intimacy.

Women, Basson argues, usually experience spontaneous sexual response only at the beginning of a new relationship or after a period of separation from their partner. The rest of the time, in everyday, established relationships female sexual desire has to be triggered to get going, rather than being spontaneous. Despite searching in vain for spontaneous desire, she writes, 'many women who are sexually functional and satisfied do not have the conventional markers of spontaneous sexual desire'.[56]

Basson says our libido is generally dormant: 'Women have a lower biological urge to be sexual for release of sexual tension'.[57] Women start out in *sexual neutrality*—receptive to being sexual but not inclined to initiate sexual activity—but the desire for intimacy prompts them to seek or accept certain stimuli to 'ignite sexual desire'. In other words, unlike men, women have to look for something to turn them on. Once they are aroused, sexual desire motivates them to continue the activity.

To women who are not happy with their lack of desire, Basson basically says, Go and find a sexual stimulus and choose to be receptive to it. She says: 'This [new] model posits a receptive type of desire stemming from arousal which itself results from the deliberate choice to find and be receptive to sexual stimuli.'[58]

On one hand this sounds quite empowering, but Basson says many obstacles confront any would-be intimacy hunter: lack of tenderness, respect, communication, or pleasure from sexual touching; undue focus on the act of intercourse itself; physical or emotional discomfort; lack of caring, consideration, safety or privacy; non-sexual distractions and other psychological factors. Quite a list.

Basson believes that where women have sexual difficulties, changes in a number of areas can make their sexual response cycle more efficient: 'Moving from a feeling of inferiority and dysfunction because spontaneous sexual neediness is rare or absent, [women] come to *accept the need for useful stimuli* and the extreme relevance of their emotional intimacy. Given that this is their driving force . . .' (italics mine).[59]

The reference to 'useful stimuli' is intriguing. Given the many obstacles to intimacy articulated by Basson, find such seems like quite a challenge. I cannot help thinking that this model maybe opens the door to pharmaceutical intervention as a means of 'useful stimuli'.

The researchers Michael Sand and William Fisher asked 110 American women which sex model suited them best: that of Masters and Johnson, Kaplan or Basson. Drum roll . . . almost equal numbers of women endorsed the Masters and Johnson model (33), the Kaplan model (30) and the Basson model (32). Another 15 women said none of the models matched their sexual functioning.[60]

What's also interesting is who found which model the most fitting . . . a sort of sexological Cinderella. The Masters and Johnson and Kaplan model was supported by women who were sexually functional, according to the Female Sexual Function Index (FSFI); premenopausal; moderately or very satisfied with their sexual relationship; and motivated to have sex in order to have sexual feelings, sensations, excitement and orgasm. The Basson model was most supported by women who were sexually dysfunctional according to the FSFI; postmenopausal; very or moderately *dissatisfied* with their sexual relationship; and who, even without physical desire, went ahead with sex for non-sexual reasons such as in hopes of feeling emotionally close.

The researchers conclude that the Basson model represents more dysfunctional and dissatisfied women's sexuality, and does not necessarily reflect normal sexual response. They believe that their overall findings emphasise the diversity of female sexual response. The 'right model', then, must draw on our life experiences. The polarity between the models of Masters and Johnson and Basson may reflect the shifting nature of our sexual response as we get older, our exposure to life's pressures, and the length of our relationships.

Will there ever be a unified theory of sex drive? It's hard to tell when so many of the researchers looking at this question are being funded by pharmaceutical giants. In a world where intellectual enquiry usually requires a financial return, models of sexual response are developed and used for diagnosis, leading to treatments. Few would question the benefits of science in treating humanity's ills, but we have to be aware of the enormous breadth of the human experience and beware of simple answers.

Sex and culture

Erica, my best friend in high school, came from Chile. She said that in her country, men often had their first sexual experience at a brothel. I found this earth-shattering. How would this affect their future, how they felt about women, their sexuality? I was astonished that this was considered normal and approved of, rather than being hidden or seen as deviant. I later learned that loss of male virginity at a brothel is common in many Latino cultures.

This had a great impact on me. I went on to study anthropology, and read about sexuality in the Middle East and Africa, in the Polynesian islands, and in my native Canada. It appeared that everything from homosexuality to infidelity, was enacted differently depending on where you grew up. The sociologists William Simon and John Gagnon gave a name to the lessons we learn about sexuality in any given culture: *sexual scripts*.[61] And it is true that much of our sexual behaviour is guided by implicit and explicit social scripts, which deem some sexual behaviours appropriate, and others perverse.

When I started my PhD, I knew what I wanted to study—young women's experience of sexuality—but I didn't know which country to focus upon. But then I started reading about the Philippines. I was riveted by its mixture of East and

West, Spanish Catholicism,[62] machismo culture, Madonna/whore attitudes and sex tourism, so I chose the Philippines as my site for fieldwork.

One of the questions I focused on was how virginity loss was viewed in the local culture.[63] Did it usually happen before or after marriage? Did it mean different things to men and women? I found that, as in the West, there was a huge double standard. Herein lies a 'truth' about human sexuality: what men do, women usually cannot. Despite the exposure of young Filipinos to modernity—higher levels of education, urbanisation, Western media, and so on—premarital sex for women is still a huge no-no. If you are not a virgin when you get married, you are considered a *disgrasyada,* a disgrace.

The most common thing Filipinas say about their virginity is that 'it is the best *gift* you can give your husband'. Others said virginity was like a mirror: if you break it, you can repair it, but it will never be quite the same. Many believed that they should marry the man to whom they lost their virginity—who else would want them?

Now, although many men in the Philippines have their first sexual encounter with their girlfriend, a significant proportion have it with a commercial sex worker. This is perceived as a rite of passage to manhood, and is referred to locally as a 'sexual baptism'. Usually a group of peers—sometimes including older men such as uncles or grandfathers—drink together, watch porn and then make their way to a brothel. Friends will often pay the prostitute to have sex with the virgin man, offering her to him as a *gift.*

Even if women save their virginity for their husband, it's very likely he will seek sex outside the marriage, either at a brothel, through casual encounters, or in the arms of a mistress, a woman who has already 'fallen'. It is not considered appropriate for a woman to ask her husband to use condoms during extramarital pursuits. Because of cultural taboos, many women look the other way. This leaves wives at risk of sexually transmitted infections and heartache.

Now, imagine if you will the reverse scenario. Imagine I told you I had done my fieldwork in Zana, a small island off the east coast of Africa. In Zana the sensuality of women is celebrated in seasonal festivals. Some women even carry small clay amulets depicting the only body part purely designed for pleasure, the clitoris. Virginity, for a young Zanan woman, is lost whenever she decides it 'feels right'. Her mother throws a party, and all the young women get drunk, look at erotica, then make their way to the local brothel accompanied by aunts and sometimes a grandmother. There, the group of friends pick the most desirable young man and pay him to pleasure the young woman. And that is that. Afterwards, the woman can have as many lovers as she pleases, and their number would be looked upon as an omen of prosperity.

Zana, of course, doesn't exist. But the story highlights how culture and gender shape our sexual practices.

Puberty rites, first sex, contraception, homosexuality, polygamy, dating, prostitution, incest, monogamy, adultery, divorce and many other things are shaped by the particular culture and time we find ourselves in. Far from being 'natural', ideas about sex and sexuality shift across cultures and across history.

We now use the term 'sexuality' to encompass sexual desire and attraction, sexual activity and behaviour and sexual identity. Our sexuality is influenced by human sexual response patterns, cultural attitudes toward sex, and our individual upbringing. Sexuality is regulated by social norms and social organisation and is linked to institutional and interpersonal power relationships related to sex and gender.[64] Sex, gender and sexuality are all 'live': dynamic, shifting in meaning and mutual interrelationship.

In 1984 the American anthropologist Gayle Rubin wrote an important essay, 'Thinking Sex', which argued that in Western societies certain sexual behaviours are rewarded, while others are punished. Under the category 'Good, Natural, Normal' she lists sex that is heterosexual, married, monogamous, procreative, non-commercial, in pairs, in a relationship, between people of the same generation, enjoyed in private, includes no pornography, involves bodies only, 'vanilla'. Under the heading 'Bad, Abnormal, Unnatural' she lists sex that is homosexual, unmarried, promiscuous, non-procreative, commercial, performed alone or in groups or in public, casual, cross-generational, includes pornography or manufactured objects, or is sadomasochistic.[65]

Certainly, what is deviant or unusual in one society may be normal in another. Polygamy was once openly practised in the US state of Utah and parts of Europe, but now isn't, although it's common in other countries, particularly in the Islamic world. Polygamy is legal in Kenya and is recognised by the courts under customary law. Homosexuality was never illegal in the French colonies, but was criminalised in all the British colonies. Intergenerational sex between males was practised in ancient Greece but is now is illegal in modern Greece, although it is common in some parts of South Asia and the Middle East. The marriage in some Asian cultures of prepubescent girls to old men would be labelled abusive if it occurred in the West. And in the modern-day West, many of us believe lust and monogamy go hand in hand!

As discussed in John D'Emilio and Estelle Freedman's 1988 work, *Intimate Matters: A History of Sexuality in America*, our sexuality fluctuates according to economics, family structure and politics.[66] The authors discuss how over the last 300 years, the role of family life in the US has radically shifted. A family-centered system based on reproduction and social stability transformed in the nineteenth century into a more romantic view of marriage, leading to our current commercialised sexuality that promises fulfillment, personal identity, and happiness through the medium of sex partnerships.

Although we are born in either male or female bodies, there is a difference between biological sex and the social construct of gender. While sex refers to biological differences, gender is based on structures of social relations related to reproduction, and the characteristics that a given culture delineates as masculine or feminine, which become part of an individual's personal sense of self.

Intersex people (also known as hermaphrodites, or people with internal/external genital discrepancy) show that biological sex is more complex than simple maleness or femaleness. Transgender people also challenge the idea of two genders—for example, the *hijra* in India and Pakistan, *tomboi*s, or *tom*s, in Thailand, and *fa'afafine* in Samoa.

Many theorists argue that sexual interaction is one of the most powerful domains in which men and women feel peer pressure to act in gender roles.

Second-wave feminism was all about a woman's right to define her own sexuality, outside of the rules of gender. Critiquing the concept that sexual pleasure was based solely in heterosexual penile penetration left open the possibility that there existed somewhere an authentic female sexuality yet to be revealed.[67] Feminist debate in the 1980s, referred to as the 'sex wars', centred on the extent of women's sexual agency, particularly in relation to issues such as pornography, sadomasochism and prostitution. Carole Vance argued that there had been an overemphasis on the *dangers* of sexuality, and that women had not been encouraged to explore their sexual pleasures.[68]

Today, immersed in a culture that glamorises sex, we find it increasingly problematic not to want it. Discrepancy in desire, arousal, orgasm or sexual pleasure can lead to a diagnosis of sexual dysfunction. All this is taking place in a climate in which the people coming up with the blueprint for sex—models of sexual normality and abnormality—are often funded by pharmaceutical companies. So now the 'low' libido many modern Western women experience as their usual state of affairs is being pathologised as a *disorder*.

6

The cover-up: 'female sexual dysfunction'

Religion once defined morally acceptable sexual conduct, but in an increasingly secular society, this task fell to medical science.

Graham Hart and Kaye Wellings[1]

The history of sexual pharmaceuticals reveals a succession of new ways to boost female desire . . . and a succession of roadblocks. At first, most treatments aimed to increase blood flow to the genitals. Then a second generation of drugs focused on upping our sex hormones. In 2004, Pfizer called off its study of Viagra (sildenafil) in women because of unconvincing results. Months later, the US Food and Drug Administration (FDA) jettisoned Procter & Gamble's testosterone patch Intrinsa, which had been linked to increased risks of heart disease and cancer. Sexy.

More recently the proposed drug flibanserin was marketed as a panacea to treat women with low desire, a pink Viagra. Considering that Viagra is one of the most popular drugs *ever*, one can only imagine the result of this second coming: a Viagra-fem-sex popping nation. After all, it wasn't all that long ago that the thought of widespread antidepressant use was like science fiction. However, after much hype the FDA rejected flibanserin in 2010, owing to questionable efficacy and concerns about side-effects.

While the effect of Viagra is essentially physical—to make the penis hard and keep it that way—increasing sexual desire in women or making orgasm easier is a more challenging endeavour. Although the FDA has approved a handheld vacuum device that increases blood flow to the clitoris, very few of the creams, patches, nasal sprays and pills produced to treat female sexual dysfunction have received government approval in the US or Australia. This, however, hasn't stopped doctors prescribing various drugs 'off-label' (see Chapter 9).

Drug companies capitalise on the unknown scope of women's sexuality and label us faulty. The Australian journalist Ray Moynihan, in his 2005 paper 'The marketing of a disease: female sexual dysfunction', published in the *British Medical Journal,* critiqued the propaganda involved in Procter & Gamble's marketing of its testosterone patch. Moynihan wrote that before the patch gained approval, the company 'unleashed a multilayered global marketing campaign', sponsoring conferences on sexual medicine, hiring sex researchers as consultants and producing a 'guide' to testosterone. This allowed Procter & Gamble to promote awareness of the 'disease' female sexual dysfunction, prompting the general public to conclude that certain drugs can target female sexual problems.[2] Moynihan quoted the psychologist Leonore Tiefer as saying: 'The product the company is selling at this stage is really the disease . . . It only has to get people talking about the condition, and present it as amenable to a drug intervention. Then it won't be seen as the company pushing its product, it will be seen as health education.'[3] Tiefer said that one of the main goals of any drug-company marketing campaign is to make people believe their complex problems are the result of a medical condition.[4] Rather than, say, life.

In his article, Moynihan also noted concerns over whether the women who took part in the testosterone patch trials even had sexual dysfunction to begin with. He reported that many of the researchers had financial conflicts of interest: at least two headed for-profit research companies that had contracted with Procter & Gamble to conduct clinical trials. Call it 'synergy', but this proves sometimes the more one discovers, the more tangled it all gets.

The German company Boehringer Ingelheim (BI) was hoping flibanserin, which it initially developed as an antidepressant, would be just the ticket to eradicate low female libido. Flibanserin affects the workings of serotonin and dopamine. A recent study found that after taking 100-mg daily doses for a month, women with 'hypoactive sexual desire disorder' (HSDD) reported an average of 2.7 additional satisfying sexual experiences a month, to a total of 4.5. The thing is, the placebo (dummy pill) had pretty much the same effect—increasing satisfying sexual experiences to 3.7 a month.[5]

Reflecting on the operational strategies of big pharma, a representative of the American New View Campaign against the medicalisation of sex told me:

> In order to create a market for their products, drug companies need to define or redefine a 'disease' so that it appears to require pharmaceutical intervention. In the case of flibanserin, this 'disease-mongering' is through BI's framing of HSDD. In lieu of FDA approval of fliban-serin, BI has already launched a million-dollar marketing campaign, using erroneous claims and pseudo-science to convince women that HSDD is extremely prevalent and from a biochemical imbalance—that their sexual desire starts in their brain and that anything low is diseased. The plan being that if flibanserin was approved, a demand for the drug would already have been created.

Ray Moynihan is also uneasy about the merging of science and marketing. Discussing this with me, he said:

> This is a huge problem . . . Almost every conference you go to, almost every education event or workshop where doctors meet, the drug companies are picking up the tab. This means the shadow of the drug company's influence hangs over so much of what goes on in medicine, and this is especially true of sexual dysfunction . . . The industry

is like a god, ever present. The pro-drug perspective is always in the room.

Who is sexually dysfunctional?

When it comes to our knowledge about female sexual dysfunction, as in who actually experiences it versus what the drug companies would have you believe, data seem to be widely inflated or completely lacking—especially from a cross-cultural perspective. Now, the main statistic flouted by researchers and drug companies alike is that the total prevalence of sexual dysfunction in Western women is 43 per cent, sending an obvious 'Mayday: most-of-us-are-sexually-numb' kind of message. This figure was announced by Edward Laumann, one of America's leading authorities on the sociology of sex, in a 1999 paper titled 'Sexual Function in the United States: Prevalence and Predictors', which was published in the *Journal of American Medical Association*.[8] However, as every divorce lawyer knows, the fine print is crucial.

The female participants in Laumann's study were classified with a sexual dysfunction if they answered yes to just *one* of seven questions—whether they had experienced a lack of desire for sex, arousal difficulties, inability to achieve climax, anxiety about sexual performance, physical pain during intercourse, not finding sex pleasurable or—wait for it—climaxing too rapidly. Not wanting sex or reaching orgasm too quickly constitutes clinical dysfunction?

What's more, most of the problems experienced by the participants in Laumann's study weren't physical, but rather associated with negative experiences in sexual relationships and general wellbeing. Also, the women weren't asked if they found their 'sexual problem' distressing, which is one of the defining criteria of sexual dysfunction according to the DSM-IV—the psychiatrists' standard reference manual. Studies that leave out the 'bothered by' component are bound to lead to inflated rates of sexual dysfunction. And another point: Laumann and some of his co-authors had links to Pfizer. Laumann has served on its Scientific Advisory Panel for well over a decade.

As Ray Moynihan notes, even though Laumann and his colleagues stated that their study method was 'not equivalent to clinical diagnosis', drug companies and other researchers have seized on this '43 per cent' statistic as a kind of Holy Grail. The figure has stuck, contributing to an overmedicalisation of women's sexuality.

Imbalanced research, write American psychologists Leonore Tiefer and Ellen Kaschak (of the New View), leads to a 'perpetually gullible, anxious, and exploitable public, the perfect market for selling magical drugs'.[7]

But before trying to fix the problem, we need to understand it. Before buying shares in whatever Love Potion No. 9 is fashionable, we need a baseline—cross-cultural data about women's sexuality and sexual satisfaction. We do not have this. What we have instead are studies about women's sexual difficulties and sexual dysfunction, which by and large are linked to pharmaceutical companies, focused on people with existing sexual health problems with little data from representative samples, or methodologically flawed.

Unsurprisingly, there's a lot of disagreement over the clinical diagnosis of female sexual dysfunction. And many women categorised as such don't believe they have a sexual problem. In a 2007 study by Michael King, for example, 38 per cent of women were diagnosed with female sexual dysfunction according to the World Health Organization's ICD-10 disease-classification criteria, but only 18 per cent of these women agreed with their diagnosis. And rates of female sexual dysfunction fell from 38 per cent to 6 per cent when women were asked if they found the problem somewhat or very distressing.[8]

Again, when women were asked what they thought was causing their sexual problems, emotional and relationship difficulties were the most common answer, not something biologically based. King writes: 'Between one half and two thirds of women in this study suggested that difficulties with their partner lay at the base of their problems. Thus, reduced sexual interest or response in women often appears to be an adaptation to stress or an unsatisfactory relationship. *Many such adaptations may be short term and not classifiable as dysfunction*.' (italics mine) This led King and his fellow researchers to surmise that whether or not a woman has a sexual problem is subjective and 'depends on the values, wishes, and sexual knowledge of the women and her partner'.[9] By the same token, classifying women's sexual problems has either 'borrowed from analogous criteria in men or depended on top-down consensus agreement by experts'. Like Moynihan and Tiefer, King concludes that 'There is concern . . . that epidemiological studies, particularly those funded by the pharmaceutical industry, report inflated prevalence rates for sexual disorders and thereby create a "need" for treatment'.[10]

Designer labels

Like fashion, defining sexual function and sexual dysfunction is dictated by trends. What is sexually 'normal' and what is sexually 'abnormal' varies across culture and time. If you were a male Roman, you might have had master–slave sexual relationship with a younger man. Believe it. Or say you were a Japanese wife in 2012 packing your husband's suitcase for a business trip. You might well slip some condoms into his luggage so that if he cheats during his sojourn, at least he will be protected. As Uwe Hartmann and colleagues note in a 2002 paper:

> ... the appropriateness of sexual behaviour are judged against the specific social and cultural norms of a given epoch. Whereas, for example, 100 years ago, a sexually interested and sensuous woman was regarded as mentally disturbed, a *lack of sexual interest* is nowadays judged as a clinical symptom requiring treatment.[11]

According to the French philosopher Michel Foucault, studies of sexual behaviour enabled mass surveillance and control of such behaviour, through public health mechanisms and self-regulation.[12] Scientific studies establish norms and standards and can leave many people feeling inadequate—when, for example, faced with stats such as the average number of times women have sex each month.

It's been hard for experts in the field to come up with an agreed definition of sexual dysfunction. As with couture, it's all in the details. The thing is, if something is just a sexual *problem* and not a *dysfunction*, there is no need for drug companies to get involved. As the investigative writer

Brian Deer notes, 'For hospital ethics committees to approve new-product trials, they must first have a disease for the product to treat. No disease, no treatment. End of story.'[15]

The current concept of 'female sexual dysfunction' arose from a number of conferences—gatherings of clinicians, researchers and drug company representatives—which sought new definitions and classifications of desire, arousal, orgasm and pain disorders.[14] These new definitions changed our global understanding of female sexuality, as they became used for diagnosis and classification of sexual disorders in the World Health Organization's ICD:10, as well as the revised edition of the *Diagnostic and Statistical Manual of Mental Disorders* (DSM-IV).

Sounds impressive, but in 1999, for example, 18 of the 19 participants in the International Consensus Development Conference on Female Sexual Dysfunction who helped create these new definitions were linked to a total of 22 drug companies. This led Roy Moynihan to call the new classification of female sexual dysfunction 'a corporate sponsored definition'.[15]

Below are the current DSM-IV definitions of female sexual dysfunctions.[16] Please do not self-diagnose—it's not 3 a.m. and you're not on Google.

Sexual Desire Disorders
Hypoactive Sexual Desire Disorder
Persistently or recurrently deficient (or absent) sexual fantasies and desire for sexual activity, as diagnosed by a clinician, taking into account factors that affect sexual functioning, e.g. age and the context of the person's life.

Sexual Aversion Disorder

Persistent or recurrent extreme aversion to, and avoidance of, all (or almost all) genital sexual contact with a sexual partner.

Sexual Arousal Disorders

Female Sexual Arousal Disorder

Persistent or recurrent inability to attain, or to maintain until completion of the sexual activity, an adequate lubrication-swelling response of sexual excitement.

Orgasmic Disorders

Female Orgasmic Disorder

Persistent or recurrent delay in, or absence of, orgasm following a normal sexual excitement phase with diagnosis based on the clinician's judgment that the woman's orgasmic capacity is less than would be reasonable for her age, sexual experience, and the adequacy of sexual stimulation she receives.

Sexual Pain Disorders

Dyspareunia

Recurrent or persistent genital pain associated with sexual intercourse.

Vaginismus

Recurrent or persistent involuntary spasm of the musculature of the outer third of the vagina that interferes with sexual intercourse.

To be diagnosed with any of these disorders, 'the disturbance must cause *marked distress or interpersonal difficulty*'. Also, the sexual dysfunction must not be 'better accounted for by another Axis 1 disorder (except another Sexual Dysfunction)' or 'due exclusively to the physiological effects of a general medical condition' or to drug abuse or medication.

Keep in mind, these problems can either be 'primary' (it's always been an issue) or 'secondary' (in the past you were satisfied with your sexual functioning, but you're not now).

Most 'female sexual dysfunctions' can be further broken down into: generalised (happens all the time) or situational (happens only under certain conditions, such as when hubby leaves his debris all around the house after you've spent the whole afternoon cleaning); organic (due to a medical disorder) or psychogenic (mental or emotional rather than physiological in origin); or, like a martini, mixed.[17]

Andrea, age 31, entrepreneur, lives in Melbourne, long-term relationship

Do you believe you have a problem with desire?

I've been struggling with this for many years and I've been able to mask it, disguise it, but then I recently connected with my partner again and I can see that if we don't deal with it it's going to be something that's quite detrimental to the relationship.

Do you have low desire?

There's so many things that I rather do than have sex. I rather eat, watch TV or read a book . . . It's not bad when it happens, I just don't feel any motivation or desire to. This has been going on for probably about eight years. Oh, God.

Would you say that it distresses you?

It doesn't distress me, it distresses my partner. There is a power in sexuality that perhaps I feel cut off from, not being able to relate that way, but I could be very happily celibate for the rest of my life.

Have you talked with somebody about this?

I spoke very briefly to a psychotherapist.

And why do you think your sex drive is low?

I'm not sure . . . I was very sexually aware at a young age, I wonder if I've just used it up? I was sexually abused at a young age. But I'm not sure if there was an impact.

. . . We talk about this for a while. It would seem that the abuse that Andrea endured is still a strong factor in her sexual and psychological health.

Do you feel passion in other areas of your life?

I'm an ardent feminist, so I do have big passions in other parts of my life.

> **Have you tried lengthening foreplay or using relaxing techniques prior to sex?**
>
> Foreplay bores me—I much rather go straight to the sex.
>
> **If there were a pill that would boost your desire, would you take it?**
>
> Of course. I remember how fun it was—that desire, how energised and revitalised it could be.

HSDD—real or fake?

Hypoactive sexual desire disorder (HSDD) is said to be the most common type of female sexual dysfunction. As just discussed, to be classified with HSDD, a woman must experience a persistent or recurrent lack of sexual fantasy and desire as recognised by a clinician. Further, it must cause *her*, not only her partner, personal distress.

A few points here.

First, distress is subjective. Having a low libido might worry us every now and then, but once we are established in a long-term relationship, and especially if children are involved, it seems to be the norm for many women—sex slides down The List. While in other times and cultures this was considered *de rigueur*, in our culture there is a big fuss about it, and women who feel this way are labelled deficient.

Our distress also relates to our partners. If the man in the picture isn't too bothered, the woman usually isn't either. But if he's so frustrated he's close to calling 'Hi-I'm-Tiffany'

147

numbers late at night, the sexual divergence may come to the forefront, causing more relationship disturbance.

In a 2006 study of women with HSDD conducted by Lorraine Dennerstein and her colleagues[18]—who included two big-pharma employees—the most frequently reported comment was that women felt they were 'letting my partner down'. You can see how this fits in with our society's current romantic ideal, which says couples should have frequent, electrifying sex forever. Asked how they felt about their low sex drive, many women said they were 'concerned', 'disappointed' and 'sad'.

Now, as for absence of sexual fantasies and desire for sexual activity being labelled as sexual dysfunction, isn't that simply the normal ebb and flow of female libido, particularly in long-term relationships, and in our DEY (Do Everything Yourself) culture?

And if doctors are to diagnose and treat female sexual 'dysfunction' properly, how exactly can they, in a standard 15–18 minute consultation, 'take into account the factors that affect sexual functioning', when sexual functioning is a complex nest of sexual, physiological, psychological and interpersonal components? At what point are they to delve into our past grievances and other issues that affect our sex life?

If we are supposed to expect such intricate, time-consuming work from our local doctor, we should also ask, how well have they done so far at managing our depression? Most doctors don't follow up thoroughly after writing a prescription, and very few discuss sexual wellbeing. Chapter 4, on pregnancy and mothering, discussed the great reluctance of doctors to talk about libido or loss of desire. Thus, leaving the complex task of sorting out what proportion of a woman's libido is physiologically inhibited versus psychosocially inhibited, and to what degree her brain should be altered to correct say, the serotonin situation, is certainly not as clear cut as that kids game, *Operation*.

Healthcare professionals are often reluctant to talk to patients about sexual health owing to limited time, lack of training, embarrassment, and the absence of effective treatment options.[19] An international survey of people aged 40 to 80 found that only 8 to 10 per cent of subjects had been asked about their sexual health during routine visits to the doctor.[220]

If a woman says she has low libido or has difficulty with arousal, clinicians will often diagnose by exclusion: looking at her hormone levels; asking if she is depressed or taking medications; considering how her desire is affected by stress or life changes. A woman may be overscheduled and thereby have little interest in sex. She may be dealing with a demanding job, or with subterranean problems in her marriage. So does the loss of libido represent normal change, such as ageing, long-term relationships, and the wear and tear of life; current circumstances, such as stress, motherhood or overall ennui; or a biological problem?

Integrating biological, psychological and cultural factors when evaluating low desire is called for.

Searching for real numbers

Researchers have introduced new tools—mainly questionnaires—to measure sexual function and distress. In a 2008 article,[21] Richard Hayes *et al.* show that prevalence estimates vary depending on the instruments used to measure female sexual dysfunction (FSD).

Indeed, the true prevalence of FSD in the general population is a contentious issue, with rates in published papers ranging from 8 per cent to 55 per cent. Sure, this may be a result of difference in the groups studied, but Hayes also had a hunch that it also had to do with the unstandardised instruments being used to measure FSD.

Dennerstein believes the very best way to determine FSD is clinical diagnosis. The second best, is with both a sexual function questionnaire (SFQ) and the female sexual distress scale (FSDS).

The SFQ is a self-report questionnaire that asks about the sexual response cycle, as well as satisfaction, masturbation, sexual problems and relationship wellbeing. Health professionals, sexologists and pharmaceutical companies use the SFQ in clinical practice, and as an endpoint in clinical trials of sex drugs. The questionnaire takes less than 15 minutes to complete. The 12-item FSDS questionnaire takes less than five minutes to fill in.

Dennerstein found that compared with the SFQ–FSDF duo, alternative instruments produced higher estimates of desire, arousal and orgasm disorders. Changing recall from the previous month to any month or more in the previous year roughly doubled the rates of all sexual disorders! Also, if sexual distress was included in the measurement, most disorders reduced by two-thirds or more. Furthermore, only a proportion of women with low sexual function reported being distressed about it: 32 per cent with low desire, 31 per cent with low lubrication, 33 per cent with orgasm difficulty, and 57 per cent with sexual pain.

In conclusion, Dennerstein stated: 'The absence of a standard, generally accepted convention for determining the presence of FSD represents a major limitation in current research. This inconsistency in outcome measures means it is very difficult to make valid comparisons between studies and populations.'[22] Too true. But how is this even to happen when debate still exists regarding what constitutes FSD, and what is the true nature of female sexual response?

Boehringer Ingelheim—daddy of flibanserin fame—in 2009 tried to solve the problem of no universally accepted instrument to diagnose women with HSDD by proposing its own:

An accurate diagnosis of Hypoactive Sexual Desire Disorder (HSDD) currently relies on a time-consuming interview with an expert clinician. Limited access to such expertise means that many women with HSDD remain undiagnosed. The Decreased Sexual Desire Screener (DSDS) was developed to provide clinicians who are neither trained nor specialised in Female Sexual Dysfunction (FSD) with a brief diagnostic procedure for the diagnosis of generalised acquired HSDD in women ... Given the scarcity of clinical experts in FSD and the increased interest in the development of pharmacological treatment for HSDD, there will be a growing need for simple diagnostic instruments that can be used in everyday practice by clinicians who are not specialised or experts in FSD.[23]

BI conducted a study in which women with HSDD were diagnosed by the screener they devised and by expert clinicians. Apparently their screener and the expert clinicians were in agreement in 224 out of 263 cases.

The Decreased Sexual Desire Screener has only five yes/no questions and a set of check boxes to rule out other problems like depression or stress.

Screeners such as this conjure up a future which is more Valley of the Nymphos than Valley of the Dolls where any nurse will be able to ask a handful of yes-or-no questions and then fill out a script for pink Viagra.

In the race to discover a sexual fortifier, scientists around the world have conducted studies to determine what percentage of women have a sexual disorder and what percentage have HSDD.

After reviewing the international literature, the researchers Avellant *et al.* conclude that the rate of female sexual dysfunction has reached . . . surprise . . . 43 per cent; and of men's, 31 per cent: 'Studies indicate a prevalence of sexual dysfunction among all women between 25 per cent and 63 per cent while the prevalence of sexual dysfunction in postmenopausal women varies from 68 per cent to 86.5 per cent.' Those are pretty f-off numbers. The authors report that loss of libido in the US ranges from 24 per cent to 31 per cent.[24]

Avellant's 2008 study of 919 Puerto Rican middle-aged women found that 40.8 per cent reported loss of libido. Keep in mind that results were procured by handing out self-administered yes/no questionnaires at health fairs. One has to wonder if the mojitos affected baseline results. Distress about loss of libido was not included. Tsk-tsk.

Suzanne West *et al.* in 2008 carried out the first study to provide a nationally representative estimate of sexual function among US women aged 30 to 70. It used self-reported outcome measures.[25] The overall prevalence of low desire was 36.2 per cent but the prevalence of HSDD once you throw in the now-mandatory distressed factor was . . . 8.3 per cent.

Findings from Australia's first large-scale national survey of sexual behaviour and attitudes were published in 2003 by Juliet Richters and her colleagues. The study of 8280 women and 8517 men found that 54.8 per cent of women and 24.9 per cent of men lacked interest in having sex. Among women, 28.8 per cent reported being unable to achieve orgasm and 27.3 per cent did not find sex pleasurable. There was no significant association between age and not finding sex pleasurable, being anxious about performance, or coming to orgasm too quickly.[29] However, the fraction of men and women reporting a sexual problem was a staggering 71 per cent (e.g., lacked interest in sex, unable to orgasm, did not find sex pleasurable, had trouble with vaginal dryness or keeping erection.)

Another Australian study explored female sexual dysfunction in 356 women of all ages, based on survey data.[27] It found that low desire was more likely to occur in women in long-term relationships; low genital arousal was more likely among women who were perimenopausal, postmenopausal or depressed and less likely in women taking hormone therapy; and sexual distress was related to depression. Women who placed greater importance on sex were less likely to experience low desire, low orgasmic function and low arousal. The authors concluded that 'Relationship factors were more important to low desire than age or menopause, whereas physiological and psychological factors were more important to low genital arousal and low orgasmic function than relationship factors.'[28] There is where big pharma believes it can . . . assist. If desire is all about relationship factors, but arousal is a physiological or psychological problem, then a pill will sort things out.

The 2001 Global Study of Sexual Attitudes and Behaviours (GSSAB) was the first large cross-cultural population survey to evaluate women's and men's sexuality. It looked at a total of 27,500 adults aged 40 to 80 years across 29 countries. To evaluate sexual dysfunction, the same sketchy do-you-come-*too*-much questions were asked, and distress was not brought up. Oh, and it was funded by Pfizer.

A 2005 Pfizer-funded study focused on the GSSAB findings from nine Asian countries: China, Taiwan, South Korea, Japan, Thailand, Singapore, Malaysia, Indonesia and the Philippines.[29] Participants included 3350 men and 3350 women. Compared to participants from Europe and North America, the Asian GSSAB respondents were more sexually conservative and less sexually active. More than 20 per cent of men and 30 per cent of women complained of at least one sexual dysfunction. Those who reported sometimes experiencing 'problems' were also labelled as having sexual dysfunction. Yikes. Furthermore, subjects who stated they did not see a doctor for their so-called dysfunction because 'I'm comfortable the way I am', or 'I didn't think it was very serious', or 'I thought it was an normal part of getting older', were deemed as lacking perception of the problem(s).

Similarly, a 2005 Pfizer-funded study of the GSSAB results from Spain found that 53.7 per cent of men and 61 per cent of women said they had not seen a doctor about their 'sexual problem' because they thought it was a normal part of ageing or they were comfortable with who they were.[30]

Is HSDD just a fancy term for low sex drive?

Are the new definitions of female sexual dysfunction, such as HSDD, advancing our understanding of women and their sexuality? Does such a diagnosis empower women to deal with the challenges they face? Speaking on behalf of the New View campaign, Rachel Liebert says:

> As an official DSM diagnosis, HSDD comes wrapped in a pathologising rhetoric that women with low desire are abnormal, broken, ill, and wrong. Through BI [Boehringer Ingelheim], HSDD is now also intimately tied to claims that women have diseased biochemistry . . . We also know from research on depression, that having one's distress attributed to a biochemical imbalance and underlying pathological condition, and being prescribed a psychotropic drug, can ultimately be very disempowering for women.
>
> In addition, the HSDD marketing deployed by BI narrows the cultural 'ideal' for the norms and expectations of women's sexuality—what is the 'right' way, what is the 'right' amount—which in turn can increase a woman's scrutiny, anxiety, and even distress, about her own desires.

It's true. If you really want to mess with a woman's head, compare her to a bunch of other women and say she doesn't measure up. This is marketing, not science.

Clinically, there are a host of factors that consistently prove to be linked to loss of desire. The 2008 study of female libido in Puerto Rico found that 'age, educational attainment, employment status, partnership status, current smoking, parity [number of children], physical activity, menopausal status with HT [hormone therapy] use and genitourinary symptoms were associated with loss of libido.'[31]

Juliet Richters and her colleagues regard the concept of sexual dysfunction as 'questionable'. They argue that most sexual unhappiness stems not from organic dysfunction but from sexual ignorance, unhappy relationships, differences between partners' sexual 'scripts', and moral quandaries about acceptable behaviour.[32]

As well, since sex is more often than not *relational* or *bidirectional*, former or current interpersonal and relationship problems, unsatisfactory overall sexual and emotional contexts, or having a lousy lover can all affect a woman's libido. Certainly, one common marker of sexual satisfaction, the female orgasm, may be elusive to women because of what Richters terms, 'inappropriate or unsatisfying sexual techniques rather than any inherent female difficulty in reaching orgasm'. She concludes, 'Something needs to change if sex is to be as satisfactory for most women as it is for most men.'[33]

In 2009, the Canadian sex expert Lori Brotto published a paper in the *Archives of Sexual Behaviour* that denounced Hypoactive Sexual Desire Disorder.[34] After reviewing the medical literature to redraft the definitions of female sexual dysfunction for the upcoming fifth edition of the *DSM*, Brotto and her team determined that: HSDD as we know it represents a misunderstanding of female sexuality; rarely fantasising about sex or feeling spontaneous desire for sex is not abnormal; problems associated with female sexual dysfunction should be long-lasting (over six months) to warrant a doctor's diagnosis; both HSDD and SAD [sexual arousal disorder] do not pay enough heed to the impact of interpersonal relationships; and the current definitions of female sexual dysfunction compartmentalise sexual problems when, in actual fact, women's experiences more often overlap. In other words, we should seriously revise everything we think we know about female sexuality.

Indeed, in all the hoopla to discover a pink Viagra, we overlook the fact that even if such a drug were somehow procured, there would still be a number of potential problems to deal with. For instance, Viagra apparently brought a lot of bedroom troubles to otherwise more-or-less happily celibate domains. After its release, women began complaining that their formerly sexually docile husbands were now sexually eager, upsetting the whole apple cart and issuing clear warning to researchers who ignore relationship factors.

According to Michael Perelman, clinicians' recent experiences with sexual pharmaceuticals—including three major medications to treat erectile dysfunction—found patient-initiated discontinuation rates of up to 50 per cent.[35] So even if a magic elixir for women were created, patient-initiated discontinuation rates would also likely be significant; relapse rates once the pharmaceuticals were discontinued may be high; and, most importantly, the long-term side effects would be unknown.

Within much sex research, there is an assumption that everyone should have the same interest in sex, and that the level of interest should be high. In actual fact, there is a wide range of 'normal'. It is our own satisfaction and our partner's that should concern us. Each woman has to decide what role desire plays in her life. Religion and culture once voiced what constitutes proper sexual behaviour: now we can thank medical science and our friendly media outlets for taking over the job. HSDD, after all, has only been a 'disorder' for the last 30 years.

Of course, I am not denying that some women suffer from inhibited sexual response and may benefit from pharmacological treatment. However, an overly medical approach to sexual behaviour downplays personal, interpersonal and psychological dynamics, as well as the historical suppression and persecution of female sexuality.

As the world becomes a denser global market, large corporations gain more power, and massive amounts of time and money are spent researching, patenting, commercialising and marketing new ideas. Result: the 'corporatisation of sex'. At a time when government funding of science and medical research is falling, research institutions and professionals rely more heavily on the corporate dollar. The medicalisation of sexual dysfunction is one example of the current trend to define variation from normal as dysfunctional, and to name a condition and then devise a treatment. And if the condition can be assessed by a GP or nurse in 15 minutes and fixed with a small pill—even better. An 'efficient supply chain'.

Corporatisation drives commercialisation, which feeds consumerism. In turn this creates a fertile environment for the medicalisation and treatment of human ailments. With something as labyrinthine as libido, consumers who are trained to take charge of their destinies via their credit cards feel empowered when presented with a range of products to choose from. Fixing low libido becomes a simple question of product choice. And we're good at that.

When examining the medicalisation of female sexuality, we need to be aware that equating sexual problems with sexual dysfunction is dangerous maths that adds up in the drug companies' favour. That said, from a clinical perspective, defining and understanding the causes of sexual dysfunction is important, and differences between the desire, arousal, orgasm and sexual-pain components of female sexual dysfunction continue to be debated in the literature. Given the complexity of female sexual function and dysfunction, additional cross-cultural studies about female sexuality are certainly warranted.

The problem with giving too much credence to women's 'dysfunctional' levels of sexual desire is that studies show that divorce or the start of a new relationship can revitalise an otherwise lethargic libido.[36] So perhaps novelty is the priceless drug? If only we could bottle that.[37]

7

Sexual zombies

Back

We try a new drug, a new combination
of drugs, and suddenly
I fall into my life again

like a vole picked up by a storm
then dropped three valleys
and two mountains away from home.

I can find my way back. I know
I will recognise the store
where I used to buy milk and gas.

I remember the house and barn,
the rake, the blue cups and plates,
the Russian novels I loved so much,

and the black silk nightgown
that he once thrust
into the toe of my Christmas stocking.

Jane Kenyon (American poet, 1947–1995)[1]

It is Saturday afternoon and the city is awash with the walking dead. Down the main street, in front of shopways, catching buses and limping in front of the hospital, come the half-living. They have torn hearts and bloody arms and skin as white as bone.

I push my pram, astonished, as hundreds of zombies pass by. It looks like the setting of a teen horror movie, but there are no cameras in sight.

I approach a young woman. She has dark hair, a masculine face, and is costumed as a mad scientist. I ask her what's going on.

'A zombie march,' she intones, shrugging.

Back home, I flip open my laptop and Google 'zombie march'. Wikipedia says they're fairly common, part of an underground phenomenon in large, especially North American, cities. Alerted through word of mouth and cyber sites such as Facebook, youths gather together as mock monsters and traipse through the city, moaning and grunting for brains. Eventually they end up at a preordained drinking establishment. Apparently some zombie marches are put on as spoof political rallies, but most, it seems, are just orchestrated to be 'anti'. Like tongue piercings.

It seems an insidious monster is creeping across the world and its pleasure lies in robbing us of our own. Once bitten, victims often experience disturbed sleep or appetite, low energy, poor concentration, and psychomotor agitation or retardation. Casualties also feel a loss of interest or pleasure, guilt and low spirits. Those so inflicted may turn to alcohol or narcotics to ease their pain. Intensity can range from mild to fatal.

The name of this monster is depression, and it affects both body and mind. This complex affliction changes how we think and feel, affecting our social behaviour, sense of wellbeing and overall drive. It can stop us taking care of ourselves and our responsibilities. And it can lead to the death of sex.

According to the World Health Organization, depression affects about 121 million people worldwide and is among the leading causes of disability globally.[2] Depressive disorders are the most disabling illnesses in Australia and play major roles in premature death by suicide, injury and cardiovascular disease.[3] Each year in the US over 17 million adults experience a period of clinical depression.[4] In Britain, depression is estimated to affect as many as one in five people at some point during their lives; at any moment in Britain, 1.5 million people aged between 16 and 75 are suffering from depression, and 2.7 million from anxiety.[5]

The stats also tell us that if you haven't experienced depression yourself, someone you care about probably has or will.

In the *Diagnostic and Statistical Manual of Mental Disorders* (DSM-IV), major depression is diagnosed if at least five of the following criteria are present during the previous two-week period: depressed mood, nearly every day during most of the day; marked diminished interest or pleasure in almost all activities; significant weight loss, weight gain, or a change in appetite; insomnia or hypersomnia; psychomotor agitation or retardation; fatigue or loss of energy; feelings of worthlessness or guilt; impaired ability to concentrate, and/or recurrent thought of death; suicide attempts.[6]

Genetics, the environment and biology can all contribute to depression. Psychological and interpersonal factors such as stressful life events (loss of a job), life milestones (children leaving home) and ongoing relationship problems can be associated with depression, as can certain medical conditions and medications.

Besides bipolar depression, depression is classified into three main types. Major depression, sometimes referred to as unipolar or clinical depression, is the most severe. It lasts two weeks or longer and may occur several times over a lifetime. Dysthymic disorder is chronic, low-grade depression persisting for over two years; *dysthymia* is a Greek word that means 'bad state of mind' or 'ill humour'. Finally there is unspecified depression, which includes a range of types. An episode of major depression that occurs after the death of a loved one is recognised as grief, not depression, and is a normal part of dealing with loss.[7]

However, although most types of depression are treatable, a benchmark 2003 study found that in many cases, in the US at least, treatment of depression was inadequate.[8] The US National Women's Health Resource Center also reported that practitioners underprescribe drugs, or keep patients on medications or dosages that aren't working for much too long.[9]

Women and depression

Depression affects almost twice as many women as men, but scientists can't really tell us why. The US National Institute of Mental Health (NIMH) says the nearly two-to-one ratio remains constant across racial, ethnic and economic lines.

Studies show that one in four women will experience clinical depression.[10]

The obvious question: what is going on?

Depression is a multifactorial disorder. While certain psychological characteristics and a family history of mood disorders predispose people to depression, numerous factors increase women's susceptibility—physical or sexual abuse, loss of social support, poverty, or a penchant for men predisposed to plonk. Hormonal changes associated with menstruation, pregnancy, miscarriage, the postnatal period, and the period around menopause also increase our risk. In other words, it would seem sorrow is our lot.

Although married men have lower rates of depression than single men, the NIMH found that married women generally get more depressed than single women.[11] And certainly women do bear most of the childcare load. In 2006, Australian men on average spent 4 hours and 29 minutes a day on recreation and leisure, 4 hours and 33 minutes a day on employment-related activities and 1 hour and 37 minutes a day on domestic activities. Australian women spent much less time on recreation and leisure (3 hours and 57 minutes), nearly twice as much time on domestic activities (2 hours and 52 minutes), and about half as much time as men on employment-related activities (2 hours and 21 minutes a day).[12] Discussing women's higher rates of depression, P. E. Bebbington writes: 'The manner in which prevalence varies by gender, marital status and involvement in child care suggests that depression may be linked to the particular things people do, and by the meaning they attach to what they do.'[13]

It's a given that not measuring up to gender roles creates dissatisfaction. Even if we temporarily fulfil our desire to be everything to everyone, we can't do so forever. There is a cost to over-functioning. It's even got a name: 'role strain'.

Pursuing Aaron Beck's 1967 hypothesis that an adverse life event can predict the onset of depression if it affects a personal vulnerability, psychologists Carolyn Mazure and P. K. Maciejewski conducted a study to see if stressful life events and cognitive style contributed to women's higher rates of depression. Although they found no difference when it came to men's and women's *exposure* to stressful life events, women were three times as likely to experience depression in *response* to stressful life events. The authors concluded that women are more sensitive to a wider array of events and thus more prone to depression. They also found that depression was linked to higher levels of 'concern about disapproval', which was three times greater in women than in men.[14]

In a 2001 study of similar focus, Kenneth Kendler and his colleagues found that stressful events were often perceived as more difficult depending on whether a man or a woman was experiencing them. Problems that caused women greater stress included housing problems, issues to do with the loss of a confidante, interpersonal problems or illness of people in their extended network. Men on the other hand reported higher rates of distress related to work problems, legal problems and, would you believe it, being robbed.[15]

Studies show that women frequently invest more in their social networks than men do. Sociologists R. Jay Turner and William Avison in 1989 developed the benchmark 'cost of caring' hypothesis, which basically argues that women show greater concern about others than men do and are thus more affected by events that affect others.[16] But this makes us liable to emotional problems associated with our relationships, and can give us a greater sense of obligation.

Some researchers believe that mental distress in both men and women is essentially a societal problem—a response, particularly, to the effects of capitalism on our daily lives. In a 2005 book, American psychiatrist Peter Kramer writes that 'depth seems so endangered and happiness so overblown, so commercial, so stupefying, that we may be inclined to cling to some version of melancholy'.[17]

Many feminists also believe that women's mental distress is essentially a societal problem—a response, particularly, to the constraints put on us by patriarchy. Discussing women's long association with 'madness', the Australian feminist Betty McLellan writes that 'without an acknowledgment of women's collective and individual oppression it would be impossible to understand the real depth of women's pain and anguish'.[18] She believes the types of oppression that especially damage women's health include violence in the home, rape, and pornography.

Sex and depression

Our mental wellbeing has an enormous impact on sexual desire. Studies repeatedly show that a depressed or anxious mind targets our sexual centre. As depression seeps into our body, the pulse of libido fades rapidly, leaving little space for desire.

Does low libido cause depression, or does depression cause low libido? The relationship between desire and depression isn't clear cut by any means, but most experts agree that if you treat the one, the other improves. Because sexual problems may exist independent of depression, all factors can nevertheless interplay, making it frequently impossible to work out the contribution of each component.[19]

People with depression, a major depressive disorder or bipolar disorder have a higher prevalence of sexual dysfunction.[20] Many people with depression suffer from disturbance in libido, arousal, orgasm/ejaculation, sexual satisfaction and sexual pleasure.[21]

The Melbourne psychologist Amanda Deeks writes that in women,

> Anxiety and depression have each been associated with decreased frequency of sexual intercourse and a reduction in sexual desire. Interestingly, depression has been found to be more significantly associated with low sexual interest than age and vaginal symptomatology. Symptoms of anxiety such as palpitations, rapid breathing, increased sweating, and depressive symptoms such as fatigue, decreased motivation and negative thoughts may all negatively impact on sexual desire.[22]

Major depression is associated with low sexual function in over 70 per cent of patients.[23] Indeed, loss of libido is reported in various studies to affect from 25 to 75 per cent of patients with unipolar depression, and its prevalence appears to be correlated with the severity of depression.[24]

A 2008 study of the relationship between loss of libido and depression among Puerto Rican women found that loss of libido *increased* as the number of depressive symptoms did. Other studies have shown that symptoms and signs of depression, such as mood instability, fragile self-esteem, worry, anxiety, and guilt, are reported more frequently by women with low desire.[25]

But for those in a dark place with no way out, science produced a cure.

Enter antidepressants

It seemed to me like this was one big Prozac nation, one big mess of malaise. Perhaps the next time half a million people gather for a protest march on the White House green it will not be for abortion rights or gay liberation, but because we're all so bummed out.

Elizabeth Wurtzel (American author and actress)[26]

Antidepressants were discovered in the 1950s, and treatment for mental distress changed forever. Given the popularity of the 'chemical imbalance' theory of depression, it's hardly surprising that drug therapy has swept us by storm.

Traditionally, mental health disorders were classified either as neurotic conditions—depression, anxiety, eating disorders, low self-esteem—or psychotic conditions. Psychotic illnesses were believed to have a biological basis, neurotic ones a more emotional one.[27] A step up, I suppose, from blaming the devil.

For decades biopsychiatry—the chemical imbalance theory of mental illness—has dominated psychiatry. Biopsychiatry looks to the brain to discover abnormalities. But disconcertingly, a lot of what we know about chemical neurotransmission comes from animal studies. This has led some to question, as sociologist Delanie Woodlock puts it, why 'drugs are given to humans who are deemed mentally "ill" with disorders that are not medically proven or even known?'[28]

Tricyclic antidepressants (TCAs) such as imipramine (Tofranil), desipramine (Pertofran), nortriptyline (Allegron), amitriptyline (Endep) and maprotiline (Ludiomil) were once the drugs of choice. These drugs inhibit norepinephrine reuptake, or both norepinephrine and serotonin reuptake. Reuptake is the reabsorption of the neurotransmitter chemical after a neural message is sent. Inhibiting this reuptake means more is available immediately outside the brain cells for neurotransmission. This helps with depression because it is thought to compensate for any lack of available norepinephrine and/or serotonin in the brain. About 30 per cent of people stopped taking these classes of drugs owing to side effects such as weight gain, fainting and headaches.[29]

Now, a new class of drugs is taking over. Current research focuses on the idea that depression can occur when neurotransmitter function is disrupted. Neurotransmitters are chemicals that carry signals from one part of the brain to the other. The main neurotransmitters that affect people's moods are serotonin, noradrenaline and dopamine. Selective serotonin reuptake inhibitors, or SSRIs, are the most popular antidepressants, with fewer side effects than tricyclics—although many of them do cause nervousness, nausea, diarrhoea and insomnia. SSRIs work by blocking reuptake of serotonin, allowing more of this neurotransmitter to remain available to the brain. SSRIs include fluoxetine (Prozac), fluvoxamine (Luvox), paroxetine (Aropax), and sertraline (Zoloft).

The antidepressant venlafaxine (Efexor) also affects the neurotransmitters serotonin and norepinephrine. The tricyclic antidepressant clomipramine (Anafranil) affects serotonin, but is not as selective as the SSRIs. Bupropion (Zyban), on the other hand, is a new antidepressant that is chemically unrelated to the SSRIs.

The WHO reports that antidepressant medications and brief, structured forms of psychotherapy are effective for 60 to 80 per cent of those affected.[30] However, the American psychiatrist Paula Clayton says: 'An anti-depressant generally has only a one-in-three chance of helping the person taking it recover.'[31]

Now, want to hear a statistic that will make your jaw drop? According to the US Department of Health and Human Services, 180 million antidepressant scripts are filled each year in the US. Of these, 90 per cent are SSRIs. (Here we are referring to prescribed medications for outpatients aged 18 to 65.) I wonder, do numbers like that represent a plague?

To get some perspective on the size of the drug enterprise, consider the following text from the Prozac website. It reports, 'Today, Prozac is one of the world's most widely prescribed antidepressants, having been prescribed for more than 40 million people in more than 90 countries, including more than 22 million in the United States.'[32]

Oh, another thing: compared to men, twice as many women are prescribed antidepressants.[33]

Delanie Woodlock, author of the 2005 paper 'Virtual pushers: antidepressant internet marketing and women', writes, 'the modern treatment for women's mental anguish is not a move towards ending women's oppression. Instead a pill is seen as the way to cure women's pain.'[34] In most countries, direct consumer marketing of antidepressants is illegal, so Woodlock says pharmaceutical companies have started to use the internet to globally market and advertise psychiatric drugs as 'happy pills'. She writes, 'Unlike advertisements for McDonald's which promote the message that their food will create happiness—for example the slogan "Come in my friend and share the happiness"—pharmaceutical companies are actually selling products that can be seen as the ultimate way to be joyful: through altering your brain chemistry.'[35]

Woodlock also points out that women are more heavily targeted in the advertising of psychiatric drugs in medical journals. Indeed, this led Ulrica Lövdahl, the head of a Swedish study, to conclude:

> . . . advertisements for antidepressants in medical journals currently construct depression as a female symptomatology, as was the case with advertisements for tranquilizers in the 1970s. This trend in drug advertising also revives the tendency towards biologicalization and overmedicatation of women's symptoms of mental distress.[36]

Sexual melancholia

We know that depression often depletes libido. Ironically, however, drug *treatment* for depression can further deplete it. Sexual dysfunction is a common side effect of taking many antidepressants, particularly the selective and non-selective serotonin reuptake inhibitors.

Although effective at treating clinical depression, *über* popular antidepressants such as fluoxetine (Prozac), paroxetine (Aropax), sertraline (Zoloft) and venlafaxine (Efexor) can have signficant sexual side effects, although this does not appear to be the case with bupropion (Zyban). Some studies have shown that moclobemide and doxepin may actually increase libido. In most cases, the greater the available dopamine the greater chance to enhance or retain sexual function in all sexual domains; too much serotonin, on the other hand, may disrupt desire and orgasmic function.[37]

For men, antidepressants can cause low libido, erectile dysfunction and difficulties with orgasm. For women they can cause orgasm difficulties and problems with vaginal lubrication.

Antidepressants, antipsychotics and their effect on libido

Medication	Libido effect	Other sexual effects
Selective serotonin reuptake inhibitors (SSRIs)		
fluoxetine (Prozac), paroxetine (Aropax), fluvoxamine (Luvox), citalopram (Cipramil), sertraline (Zoloft)	decrease	anorgasmia (unable to orgasm), delayed ejaculation, erectile dysfunction/decreased vaginal lubrication
escitalopram (Lexapro)	unknown	ejaculatory disorder
Monoamine oxidase inhibitors (MAOIs)		
phenelzine (Nardil)	decrease	erectile dysfunction, delayed orgasm in men and women
moclobemide (Amira)	increase	unknown
tranylcypromine (Parnate)		

Medication	Libido effect	Other sexual effects
Tricyclics (TCAs)		
imipramine (Tofranil)	decrease	erectile dysfunction, delayed orgasm in men and women
clomipramine (Anafranil)	decrease	anorgasmia, abnormal ejaculation, erectile dysfunction. one of the side effects is delayed ejaculation; because of this men are using it off-label. On the street the drug is referred to as 'the bomb'
amitriptyline (Endep)	decrease	unknown
doxepin (Deptran)	increase	unknown
desipramine (Pertofran), nortriptyline (Allegron), maprotiline (Ludiomil)	unknown	unknown
5-HT Modulators		
mirtazapine (Avanza)	decrease	delayed orgasm/ejaculation, anorgasmia/no ejaculation, erectile dysfunction/decreased vaginal lubrication
Mixed reuptake inhibitors and others		
bupropion (Zyban)	increase possible	none
venlafaxine (Efexor)	decrease	erectile dysfunction/decreased vaginal lubrication, abnormal orgasm, anorgasmia/no ejaculation, delayed orgasm/ejaculation
reboxetine (Edronax)	no change	
Antipsychotics		
haloperidol (Haldol, Seranace), thioridanzine (Mellaril, Aldazine), risperidone (Risperdal)	decrease	anorgasmia, erectile dysfunction, painful ejaculation

* This table is compiled from a number of papers, most noteworthy: Philips and Slaughter (2000), Werneke (2006) and Hollon (2003). Not all brand names are listed.

According to a 2008 study, sexual dysfunction is estimated to occur in 30 to 70 per cent of men and women treated for major depression with first- or second-generation antidepressants.[38] Rates of antidepressant-induced sexual dysfunction in the psychiatric literature are much higher, some approaching 70 to 80 per cent.[39] A 1997 study found that almost 50 per cent of patients surveyed before and after taking the SSRI antidepressants fluoxetine (Prozac), paroxetine (Aropax), fluvoxamine (Luvox), citalopram (Cipramil) and sertraline (Zoloft) experienced a decline in libido.[40]

Men report higher rates of antidepressant-induced sexual dysfunction, but women describe greater severity.[41] It is thought that women experience more side effects from antidepressant medication because their body-fat-to-muscle ratio is different, or possibly owing to hormonal effects. Thus, women may need a lower dose of antidepressant to reduce unwanted side effects.

Suffering with both low sex drive and depression, a 39-year-old mother of two said, 'I don't think an antidepressant changes your life. It doesn't make you happy or put someone on the couch beside you. It doesn't help you make friends. Yes, it gets you out of the gutter, but is it really addressing the issue of low sex drive? I think it's more important to talk about it, get your partner involved. I don't think a pill is going to make it all better. There's too much happening in a woman's brain to have the whole situation fixed by a pill.'

Recent clinic-based research also suggests that, despite effective treatment, sexual difficulties that depressed women experience often persist. A 2004 study reported that a year after psychotherapy treatment with or without antidepressants, recurrently depressed women continued to experience sexual problems.[42]

Aside from depression, other unwanted side effects of antidepressants may include restricted emotional receptiveness, reactivity and emotional withdrawal, which can lead to relationship problems.[43] Anthropologist Helen Fisher explores how drugs like fluoxetine (Prozac) may hinder our ability to fall and stay in love. Certain antidepressants, she argues, sabotage the process of attachment by altering hormone levels in the brain.[44]

One study found that 80 per cent of women don't discuss the adverse sexual effects of their antidepressants with their doctor.[45] And many doctors still don't talk about drug effects on sexual wellbeing with the patients to whom they are prescribing drugs. This is such a waste.

It appears getting your meds right is the modern-day equivalent of getting an accurate star chart. However, if the medication you or your partner is on is interfering with your sexual relationship, it might be possible for you and your doctor to work together to find a better arrangement.

In some cases it is possible to slightly lower the dosage. Under medical supervision, you may be able to reduce your dose while retaining the positive effects of the drug. For instance, this is reported to work with fluoxetine (Prozac).[46] However, reduction of antidepressants can possibly lead to relapse or recurrence of depression.[47]

If lessening dosage isn't appropriate or doesn't work, it may be possible under medical supervision to switch to another antidepressant that has less impact on sexual function. Non-serotonergic antidepressants, which have fewer sexual side effects, include bupropion and reboxetine, or mirtazapine.[48] Bupropion shows a low incidence of sexual dysfunction and may improve sexual desire in depressed patients.[49] Note, these drugs have other side effects and switching drugs is rarely a straightforward process.

Alternatively, to increase sex drive some experts suggest adding other medications to those you're already on. There is conjecture that yohimbine and amantadine could be helpful as possible antidotes to antidepressant-induced sexual dysfunction.[50] Your doctor might suggest a daily regimen, or recommend that you take the particular drug prior to sexual activity. Some doctors may advise timing antidepressant use to lessen its effect on libido. With Zoloft and Anafranil, for example, it may be possible to take your daily dose close to the time you would normally finish having sex.[51]

Some research shows that selective phosphodiesterase type 5 inhibitors (PDE51s), including Viagra (sildenafil), given to women with antidepressant-induced sexual dysfunction can amplify their *arousal*[52]—increasing engorgement, clitoral responsiveness, and lubrication—and thereby assisting women in antidepressant treatment adherence.[53] But, the thing is, it doesn't help increase *desire*. Not having received government approval, PDE51s are currently used on women off-label, for reasons not listed in the 'indications for use'. Those who prescribe Viagra suggest it can be taken 30 to 60 minutes prior to sexual activity.

Alternatively, you could consider a 'drug holiday'.[54] With Aropax and Zoloft it may be possible to have one or two days each week drug free, restoring sexual function without losing the efficacy of the antidepressant. (Note: drug holidays can put you at risk of serotonergic discontinuation syndrome with withdrawal symptoms including flu-like symptoms, sensory and sleep disturbances, anxiety and or agitation.[56]) Or, if there is any way possible, you could, *under doctor supervision*, stop taking meds altogether and seek the help of a psychologist or sex therapist.

Depression is not completely understood and the causes of depression in an individual are usually multilayered. Are antidepressant drugs the ultimate solution to our collective malaise? Of course not. But they are helping a lot of people.

Although images of sexual vitality are ablaze in the media, many of our bedrooms and bodies are cold. Although we might appear interested on the surface, and work to appear *desirable*, deep down where psyche and libido reside, it's another story. Given that women have more major depression, more antidepressant-induced sexual dysfunction and use more SSRIs,[57] it is no wonder that our sexuality is in crisis. If depression or antidepressant use is robbing you of your desire, devise a plan to steal it back.

8

Libido and the ageing body

It's official: the baby boomers are retiring. In 2009 it was estimated that there were 39.6 million Americans aged 65 or older, and by the year 2030 this number is expected to reach 72.1 million.[1] In the last two decades, the fraction of Australians aged 65 years and older has increased by 23 per cent; in Europe the proportion of people over 60 is expected to grow by 50 per cent over the next 30 years.[2]

Now, the baby boomer generation has never been known for its passivity or acceptance of mainstream norms. After all, they're the ones who burned their bras and had vagina-viewing circles. They are currently challenging stereotypes about ageing and finding new ways to do old well.

Ageing is more than a biological process. All organisms age, but what makes humans unique is that we alone are aware of our ageing and can anticipate its consequences. As such, ageing brings a profound shift of identity, shaped by the culture we live in, the individual life we have grown into, and by gender and class.

For women, mid-life is more than the cessation of menses and associated bodily changes. What it's really about is *transformation* in many areas of our life. Our family, intimate relationships, employment, social life, feelings about appearance, health and such small matters as the meaning of life all undergo radical change. Not to mention our libido.[3]

English scholar Peter Laslett suggested that human life passes through four 'ages':

- *the first age*—childhood and adolescence, characterised by dependence, immaturity, education and socialisation . . . the good old days when people looked after us
- *the second age*—young to middle adulthood, a time of independence, maturity, responsibility and partnership . . . (or not)
- *the third age*—mid-life and old age, characterised by the quest to 'make it', fulfilling personal goals, dreams and life plans
- *the fourth age*—advanced old age, described as a period of dependence, bodily decay, possible widowhood, followed by entry to the necropolis.[4]

The thing is, Laslett's ageing theory doesn't give much time to culture or gender so a bunch of other sociological theories about ageing have tried to redress this.

For example, in the 'mask of ageing' theory, the ageing body masks the true, youthful person inside and so to try to transcend ageing we adopt 'age-resistant regulatory practices'. Like dyeing out grey.[5] But there's an assumption here: that ageing is about decline and loss, when for many people, this is not the case.

Karen Ballard and her colleagues argue that ageing occurs in two simultaneous ways: publicly and privately. *Public ageing* begins early in the life course, relates to our appearance, and is determined and monitored through social interactions. *Private ageing* occurs later in the life course and is determined by an individual's evaluation of their health status.[6]

Robert Atchley's 'continuity' theory sees ageing as an evolutionary process where self and identity are simultaneously continuous *and* changing.[7]

American ageing expert Susan Sherman believes people feel a certain age based on their chronological age, their health and the role transitions they've experienced (in terms of work, parenting, grandparenting and marital roles), and in relation to their peers.[8] In other words, choosing to be friends with *Playboy* bunnies or the local knitting group will help define how old you feel.

Role change is a big mid-life identity marker. For example, the reduced demands associated with children leaving the 24-hour mum-and-dad hotel or becoming a grandparent can cause emotional upheaval in our lives. The crossover into 'elder' can be fraught with identity uncertainty. Questions arise about what is lost, what is gained, and how to spend the precious time we have left most wisely and most pleasurably.

Age, it seems, also has to do with class. A 2003 study by the American sociologist Anne Barrett found that mid-life women from lower socioeconomic backgrounds tended to report feeling older earlier than middle or upper-class women.[9] Who, we guess, have more time for things like Pilates and organic lettuce.

During their mid-life, women often find themselves in the 'sandwich generation'—caring for the generations either side of them, both their offspring and their ageing parents. Although some women suffer from 'empty nest' syndrome, others suffer from the reverse—the recent trend for adult children to move in and out of their parents' homes as they feel the need.

Karen Ballard found that women become aware of their physical ageing when they're about 40.[10] A sense of ageing becomes more pronounced through comparison with peers, through comparison with images of themselves when younger, 'self-monitoring' and—worse yet—through constant exposure to mass media that glorifies youthfulness.[11]

Now, ageing in our culture has a pretty bad rap and traditionally has been associated with invisibility and loss—loss of youth, loss of beauty, loss of fecundity. Research shows that women are under more pressure than men to maintain a 'youthful' appearance and are perceived as older sooner than men.[12] Older women are often seen as asexual and unattractive; ageing men are often regarded as sexy and wise.[13] Other researchers believe that negative images of ageing are largely targeted at women, who, swayed by social pressure, become compelled to maintain a 'youthful' body.[14] To retain status and power, many women actively work to 'look after themselves' and deny the signs of ageing.[15] Thus diet, exercise, fashion and cosmetics become imperative.[16]

I suppose this may challenge assumptions about age being associated with decline, but it also fuels the whole merry-go-round. Can't we age on our own without the weight of beauty propaganda? Where is women's space to simply be, to no longer compete? Surely, after all the years of caring, loving, struggling and hard work, we deserve this. Some women, as we will see in later interviews, through ageing liberate themselves from these cares.

Interestingly, a number of researchers have found that women who subscribe to traditional patriarchal notions of women as wives and caretakers, and of the limited attractiveness and sexual potential of older women, are more likely to internalise a negative self-concept as they age.[17] *But we can actively resist and challenge the notion that to age is to decline, and that to age is to lose our sexual vitality. To age is to change—to discover new sides of ourselves and new forms of pleasure.* Indeed, as Melbourne researcher Narelle Warren writes, many women experience this time as a period of personal growth, consolidation and freedom from old roles and responsibilities.[18]

Ageing gives us another surprise. Often a new sensuality is found in finally having time to focus on what gives us pleasure. As such, our later years can be a time of renewed or redirected desires.

Menopause

And so from where menses starts—visiting a young girl with its purple blood, bringing her towards her older sisters, towards uncertain desires—menopause ends, leaving a grown woman with a life lived behind her, and the feeling of a new, somehow different future.

When I was pregnant, the sixteenth of my weekly internet pregnancy updates ('this week your baby is the size of an avocado') told me the seemingly impossible: that within my baby's tiny ovaries millions of eggs were already forming.

We are organic beings. Our bodies are designed to grow, to mate, to copulate like sun-gods and harvest and reproduce. Our bodies are designed to nurture, to hold children, lovers, brothers and sisters. To work, to produce, to create and build. And, just as inevitably, our bodies will gradually atrophy as we approach our earthly end, all the while hoping we are leaving something tangible behind, that our footsteps somehow mattered.

While individuals have the power to shape their own life course, it is predominantly the job of culture to map ways for its members to make sense of these distinct periods of life. Different cultures, and indeed different eras, use their own maps to chart the seas of our social roles, constructing guidelines about what is expected from their members across the lifespan.

In the past, many cultures mapped both menarche and menopause as major life transitions. The shift from little girl or 'maiden', to reproductive woman or 'matron', and then to older woman or 'crone', marked a woman's experience in the world into three distinct spheres. Being an older woman had its own divinity, its own power, as the many myths surrounding the crone tell us. Despite the Walt Disney depictions, historically 'the crone' wasn't an old ugly woman with an assortment of warts and spells. Rather, she represented women's wisdom after the beauty of youth fades; she possessed magic, healing, knowledge, female autonomy and strength. She was a force to be reckoned with.

This tripartite division of a woman's life also plays out in modern times. The end of fertility is often referred to as the 'third age'. In the US in the next two decades, almost 40 million women will experience menopause. And Western women can now expect to live an average of 82 years—long enough that one-third of their life is spent post-menopause.[19] So it is important for us to explore the sensuality, pleasure and power of this terrain.

Menopause can be seen as a rite of passage—accompanied by physical and social changes—through which women must pass before entering the next stage of their lives: the older woman. For some, this conversion is met with great ceremony and significance, but for most of us in consumerist societies it is devalued.

In Western culture, menopause has symbolised the end of youth, and thus the beginning of decline: loss of youth, fertility, attractiveness, libido, social worth, value, good health, hormones, calcium and natural hair colour. Thankfully women and men alike are challenging such assumptions and living rich, dynamic lives despite their biological age. Narelle Warren explains that menopause is an evasive concept—meaning different things between and within cultures, depending on factors such as gender, age and social position. Menopause is simultaneously a social and physical experience, both cultural and biological. So if we were playing *Scrabble*, it'd get a lot of points.

From a biological perspective, our ovaries have a finite number of eggs. As the end of that supply approaches, the natural female sex hormones that regulate our ovulation and menstruation, oestradiol and progesterone, shift. In the few years leading to the final menstrual period, hormone levels can fluctuate dramatically, commonly resulting in menopausal symptoms. Hormone levels eventually decrease, menstruation stops, and menopause is reached. Menopause is generally defined as occurring after one year of continuous amenorrhoea (lack of menstrual bleeding).

Early menopause is when the final menstruation occurs before the age of 45. When the uterus is surgically removed in a younger woman (hysterectomy), her periods will cease permanently and she will technically be infertile, but as long as at least one of her ovaries is still functioning, she will not have reached menopause. But where a woman's ovaries are removed (oophorectomy), even if her uterus is intact, she will immediately be in 'surgical menopause'. Early and premature menopause can also occur naturally when hormone levels decrease, or chemically after chemotherapy or radiation treatment.

The timing of menopause is unique to every woman, although you're likely to experience it roughly around the same time as your grandmother, mum or sister did. Most women stop menstruating completely between the ages of 50 and 51, although menopause can occur as early as 35 or as late as 60.

Oestrogen is significantly reduced during the menopausal transition. Oestrogen is the primary female sex hormone and is manufactured mostly in the ovaries. It is required for the development of female sexual and reproductive organs and to maintain the female genital tissues, such as the vagina and clitoris. During the menopausal transition, progesterone is also reduced. Testosterone is a little more complicated. It is important in maintaining libido, orgasm and sexual function. Total testosterone and androstenedione start to decline in the late/mid reproductive years and circulating levels continue to decrease with advancing age.[20] Levels of circulating androgens in women at age 45 are half those of women in their 20s.[21] But since testosterone declines in women *prior* to menopause, women in their late reproductive years are just as likely to have low testosterone as women in their early menopausal years.[22] Decline in testosterone can also be sudden, such as in the case of loss of function or removal of ovaries.

Other physical ailments associated with menopause aren't exactly aphrodisiacs . . .

Vaginal dryness and irritation

Vaginal dryness and irritation is a common complaint of both menopausal and perimenopausal women. Generally, with age, blood flow to all regions decreases, which results in thinning of the vaginal walls, atrophy of the vaginal smooth muscles and less lubrication during sex. Intercourse can range from uncomfortable to painful (dyspareunia), and can sometimes cause spotting or light bleeding. Because of this, women often avoid intercourse, which can lead to further atrophy, which can worsen dyspareunia and result in performance anxiety and overall loss of libido.[23]

Clitoral and other changes

Clitoral changes resulting from aging include shrinkage, reduced engorgement during arousal and reduced responsiveness. Decreased muscle tension may increase the time to orgasm and diminish the peak. Contraction of the uterus with orgasm may also become painful with advancing age.[24]

Urinary incontinence

When oestrogen begins to drop, the pelvic floor muscles weaken and make bladder control more difficult.

Fatigue, mood swings and depression

Hot flushes, night sweats and insomnia can leave a woman tired and irritable. Changes in mood and sleep patterns can also exacerbate painful sex. Many menopausal women are diagnosed as having mild or major depression. Postmenopausal women are considered to be at increased risk of depressive mood.[25] After reviewing recent long-term studies, Ellen Freeman concluded that the chance of depressed mood during menopausal transition is 30 per cent to three times greater than during premenopause.[26]

Change in body shape

Many women gain weight between the ages of 35 and 55, usually around the abdomen—often referred to as 'the middle-aged spread'. Women gain weight at menopause because of complex changes in our biochemistry. Rather unsurprisingly, given our cultural fixation with slimness, association has been found between weight gain and depression in mid-life.

The medicalisation of menopause

In the West, biology or medicine is, without a doubt, the dominant way of framing the experience of menopause.

Medicalisation refers to treating a *natural process* as though it were a *medical condition* requiring intervention—similar to women's fluctuation of desire being treated as sexual dysfunction, or women's ageing requiring cosmetic procedure. Likewise, the biomedical model focuses on menopause in terms of managing symptoms and the risk of osteoporosis (in particular), heart disease (including stroke) and Alzheimer's disease, all of which are claimed to be managed by hormone replacement therapy.

The medical model of menopause greatly influences women's expectations and experiences. From a biomedical view, menopause is understood as a pathological condition caused by oestrogen deficiency; it's common for medical researchers, service providers and drug companies to define menopause as a hormone deficiency condition resulting from ovarian 'failure'. The pharmaceutical industry is certainly a driving force in this process. Many studies pertaining to hormones are sponsored by, you guessed it, pharmaceutical companies, which can arguably bias the way studies are conducted and interpreted.

Menopause is a natural process, part of the life course of the human female, and not a disease or a disorder. That's not to say some of the symptoms aren't seriously aggravating. And not to say that getting treatment for symptoms you find seriously aggravating is in any way inappropriate (for discussion about Hormone Replacement Therapy (HRT), see chapter 9). Menopause can be challenging and many women find themselves anxious or even scared about going through the transition. For others, menopause is a happy, exciting time in their lives: no longer bound by periods, or under the same influence of hormones, they can now live for the first time without the worry of unwanted pregnancy.

From a biomedical perspective, the menopausal transition involves three distinct stages.

- Premenopause—when women menstruate and ovulate regularly; women's fertile life.
- Perimenopause—the first stage of menopause, when ovulation is unpredictable because ovarian production of oestrogen slowing down; irregularities occur in the length, flow or patterning of menstruation. Perimenopause begins 2–8 years before the final cessation of menstruation, and persists for one year after the final menses. Fluctuating oestrogen and progesterone levels will probably cause some menopause symptoms, such as hot flushes, night sweats and mood swings, with the dial mysteriously stuck on 'irritability'.
- Postmenopause—begins when 12 full months have passed since the last menstrual period. By this juncture a woman's hormone levels have changed significantly. The ovaries have begun to shrink, but still produce some hormones, although not oestrogen or progesterone. Because oestrogen is also converted from other hormones, such as DHEA in fatty tissue, there is still oestrogen in the body.

North American data, based on women's self-reports, demonstrate that the menopausal transition often lasts much longer and moves in a less linear fashion than the biomedical model above.[27]

The biomedical model is further weakened if we look at cross-cultural research. For instance, anthropologist Margaret Lock's 1998 comparative study of Japanese, American and Canadian women's experiences found that women from different cultures reported different menopause symptoms. Hot flushes were common with North Americans, while Japanese women rarely experienced hot flushes or headaches, but did report shoulder stiffness.[28] In fact, women in some non-Western cultures seemingly don't 'suffer' through menopause. Fascinatingly, Rajput women in India[29] and Mayan women from South America[30] report no menopausal symptoms at all. Anthropologist Yewoubdar Beyene discovered that in cultural groups where women's ageing is not associated with a loss of status, menopause was not experienced as a difficult, negative event. That said, in most cultures women do suffer from some menopausal symptoms.

In a recent survey by Pharmacia Corporation, 1200 women were questioned to see how ethnicity impacted upon perceptions of menopause. African women were the most optimistic. Caucasian women were the most anxious. Asian women were more muted about symptoms and Hispanic women were the most stoic.[31]

Another 1999 study compared the menopausal experience of 70 Filipinos and 70 Australians (median age, 47).[32] Although the physical experiences were found to be quite similar, psychologically they were poles apart. Filipino women were more positive, the majority reporting that they felt only minor if any psychological difficulties. Most were looking forward to the joys of old age—being loved and respected by the family and the wider community.

About one-quarter of the Australians, on the other hand, found it difficult to come to terms with the ageing process and reported irritability, depression, fear, loneliness, mood swings, unhappiness and loss of self-esteem, respect and admiration. Much of this grief stems not from a loss of fertility but from fear of ageing in a culture that venerates teenagers.

International research has shown that women experience a plethora of perplexing so-called menopausal symptoms—such as dry eyes, discomfort peeing, nervous tension, tingling in the hands and feet, chest pain upon exertion, sore throat, bladder infections, and a dry nose or mouth. But epidemiological data suggest that very few of these or other symptoms are menopause-based. Most are actually related to biological, cultural, social, spiritual, medical or psychological factors.[33]

Indeed, beyond changes in menstrual bleeding and the experience of hot flushes/night sweats, a number of researchers believe that symptoms have been attributed to menopause when in actual fact there is a lack of evidence that they are distinct from general ageing or other problems that occur in midlife.

Ellen Freeman and her colleagues looked at whether menopausal symptoms increased through the menopausal transition.[34] After studying 404 American women longitudinally for nine years (by interviews, questionnaires, menstrual bleeding dates and early follicular hormone measures) they reported in 2007 that the prevalence of hot flushes, aches, joint pain and stiffness, and depressed mood *increased* during menopause stages and were related to shifting hormones. Poor sleep, decreased libido and vaginal dryness, however, did *not* appear to be associated with the menopause transition. Interestingly, high stress was closely linked to menopausal symptoms, including decreased libido and vaginal dryness. Also, reproductive hormone levels and fluctuations, particularly of oestradiol, were linked to menopausal symptoms. Freeman found that depressed mood increased in the early menopausal transition.

In a 2010 study Freeman looked at whether women are at risk of getting depression during the menopausal transition and how this may be related to changing hormones. She found that although many women report dysphoric (unhappy) mood, poor sleep, aches and joint pains, and changes in cognition and libido around menopause, it is controversial whether these symptoms are associated with the hormonal changes of ovarian aging.[35] Further research is called for to better understand how hormonal shifts—particularly of androgens—impact our experience of menopause.

If, as anthropological studies have indicated, no universal menopausal symptoms exist—and the symptoms women do experience are related to the culture they're raised in, then menopause is physically, psychologically and socio-culturally mediated.

Jean Enrique Blumel and his colleagues (2004) discovered that family problems can exacerbate menopausal symptoms.[36] Support from family and community, then, is especially important for menopausal women.

So what we now know of menopause is that a gap exists between the biomedical model and what real women experience, and that what real women experience is different depending on which culture they've grown up in. You can see that it's the same story for women's sexuality—science says one thing, but women's lives reveal a much more complex and nuanced picture.

Sex and ageing

We know from the earlier chapter on sex prime that peak hormones don't necessarily translate to peak sexual performance. It isn't like the Olympics. In fact, many of us never reach our full sexual potential: 'the ability to be comfortable in one's body, suspend time and communicate through the skin'.[37]

Sex, they say, is sense-driven. Unfortunately our senses deteriorate as we age, and not only our sight, hearing, and sense of taste. Numerous studies have shown that we also experience a loss of tactile sensitivity—we may encounter reduced or changed sensations of pain, vibration, cold, heat, pressure and touch.[38]

Like much about women's sexuality, little is known about women's sex drive and functioning as we age.[39] Although the vast majority of studies show that sexual function declines as we get older,[40] a number have also shown that women retain sexual activity and satisfaction as they age. Basically, we don't know why sexual function declines for most women but not in others, and there certainly isn't consensus about what constitutes 'normal' female sexuality across the lifespan.[41] The fact that there are few long-term studies on the topic doesn't help.

There are numerous reasons why sexual desire can decrease as men and women age, including changes in physical and mental health,[42] retirement, diminished income, divorce, unresolved anger, separation from loved ones, medical illnesses, major depression and some medications[43], including SSRI antidepressants. For women in particular, factors include: hormonal and physiological changes associated with menopause, the availability of a partner interested in and capable of sexual activity,[44] feelings of low self-esteem, insecurity and loss of femininity,[45] length of a relationship, boredom with a relationship, overall feelings for a partner, and widowhood.[46] Research indicates that women's desire levels are often linked to their relationship, whereas for men this is not always the case.[47] Laura Carpenter (2009) suggests that lower levels of sexual satisfaction in older age stem from generational differences more than from ageing itself.[48] Indeed, as women age, their priorities may shift, and sex may not be given the same centrality. Other research shows that previous levels of sexual function are the most important predictor of current sexual activity.[49]

Although women's ethnic background and cultural upbringing greatly influence their later-in-life sexuality,[50] little research has explored sexual function in racially and ethically diverse women.[51] However Alison Huang's 2009 American study of 1977 middle-aged and older women (white, African-American, Latina and Asian) found that self-reports of sexual desire, activity, and satisfaction varied according to race and ethnicity.[52] Nancy Avis's study (2007) also showed a number of racial and ethnic differences: African American women reported higher frequency of intercourse; Chinese and Japanese women engaged in fewer different manifestations of sexuality than Western women and their sexuality was more linked to procreation.[53]

The sexual changes associated with menopause were covered earlier in this chapter, but men also face a number of age-related sexual changes. In mid-life, men begin to experience changes in their hormone levels, blood flow, libido, sensitivity and ability to ejaculate. Age-related changes include lowered testosterone levels, decline of sperm production, diminished force of ejaculations, increased size of the prostate gland, slower development of excitement and erections, difficulty maintaining erections for longer periods prior to ejaculation, and less frequent ejaculation.[54]

Illness can affect our sexuality, and as we age, we're more likely to experience disabling conditions and illnesses that may affect our sexual response, ranging from diminishing energy or strength to major problems such as cardiovascular disease, diabetes, stroke, arthritis, cancer, coronary disease, Parkinson's or Alzheimer's disease, recovery from surgery, and the side effects of medication.

Melinda, age 48, lives in Melbourne, owns a marketing business, and has a long-term partner. She was diagnosed with breast cancer last March. She started chemotherapy, which brought forth menopause. Describing her sexual relationship, she said:

> We got together eight or nine years ago and for the first 12 months were very sexually intimate, and then he lost *all* interest, and I didn't really do much about it. I didn't want to look like a fool. I talked to him, but I didn't push any action to get things going again. He said he didn't know why. Despite this, he's the love of my life. We just went a number of years without sexual intimacy.

With the diagnoses, after twelve weeks of treatment, we went away for a week, and yes, we had one brief encounter, which was lovely. Afterwards, I asked him, 'What was it like not having breasts?' And he went, 'Oh yeah!' He didn't notice I didn't have the girls in!

I asked Melinda whether cancer changed how she felt about herself as a woman.

I feel like superwoman. I have a great sense of pride in myself. In my early 40s, I thought, god, this is middle age. I was feeling ugly, overweight and old. I was down all the time, I was angry most of the time and then I had a huge wake up call. None of that shit matters at all.

She also discovered new pleasures:

I've written a children's book. I've taken up painting . . . My marketing business, well, I started tweeting last year, updating my website from bed with chemo, and now I have a waiting list of clients. My partner says it's because I'm so much more confident now.

And was she able to resolve the sexual discrepancy that she described earlier?

I don't think I did. I was angry with him underneath. We had originally met when I was in my early 20s and he in his 30s. I had an instant crush. We were mates for about a year. He just wasn't interested. I tried to act real cool. We kept in touch. We moved on. I married someone else; he married someone else. We finally got together when I was in my early 40s. And he was very interested.

It was terribly sexual and romantic when we were living in different states. But then I moved in with him and it all stopped. And when it stopped it made sense, because it was the same as he was back then. That really gave my identity a bit of a bash and in a way reinforced what I already thought. I didn't think, 'This is unusual, someone doesn't want me.' I thought, 'Of course.'

The psychological effects of illness can also diminish our libido, especially if we have, or our partner has, a life-limiting or life-threatening illness. If the illness affects self-esteem or alters body image drastically (such as a with mastectomy), sexual function—along with a hell of a lot of other things—will likely be disrupted. Poor self-image as a 'sick person' can also play a role.

Illness often changes the psychosexual dynamic of a couple. The equilibrium of the emotional connection changes when one or both parties becomes ill—for instance, those who were previously independent can become highly dependent. The overall stress and exhaustion involved in caretaking can understandably spoil desire.

Life outlooks influence sexual outlooks. Some view retirement and children leaving home as the end chapter of a life, and this can cause depression and a sense of displacement and purposelessness. Others view it as open terrain, when the 'self' finally gets prime real estate.

Men and women are living longer, healthier lives than in any other time in history. Many older couples have sexually fulfilling lives. It's important too to distinguish between the 'age' of a relationship and the age of partners in a relationship. An older woman, for example, could be in the throes of a new relationship, in a long-term satisfying relationship or a long-term dismal relationship, or she could be single. Because older people are often stereotyped as asexual, health care providers don't necessarily talk about sex with their elderly patients, and many nursing homes and elderly-care residences give scant consideration to sexuality or privacy,[55] although thankfully this is changing.

Viagra's accomplishment of tendering a second life to men by giving them a reliable penis stimulated research into later-life sexuality and also drew welcome attention to the sexuality of postmenopausal women, a formerly soggy research terrain. Nevertheless, much research on older people medicalises sexual issues, focusing on the negative impact of age.

In a 2007 study, John DeLamater and Sam Moorman[56] aimed to counter these attitudes by collecting data on diagnosed illnesses, treated illnesses, sexual desire, sexual attitudes, partner circumstances and sexual behaviour from 1384 people aged 45 and older. They discovered that many of the medications their subjects were being prescribed slowed the autonomic nervous system, thus reducing responsiveness and sensitivity to stimulation. These medications were believed to interfere with the ability to sustain sexual thought and fantasy. His general findings also supported a previous DeLamater study which found that older people who lack a sexual partner for a lengthy period often 'drift into a state of sexual disinterest'.[57] Having interviewed many single older women, I tend to agree. Women often 'turn off' their interest as a coping mechanism—no longer wanting sex prevents frustration about being alone.[58]

Surprisingly, however, DeLamater and Moorman also found that diagnosed illnesses and treatments did not seem to impact upon the frequency of sexual activity. Rather, it was sexual *attitudes* that affected the frequency of sex. Positive attitudes about sex and having a physically satisfying relationship were strongly associated with greater frequency of sexual behaviours in both men and women.

Likewise, a 1998 National Council on Aging survey of 1300 Americans over the age of 60 showed that sexual activity plays an important part in the relationships of older people. Forty-eight per cent reported having sex at least once a month. Of these respondents, 79 per cent of men and 66 per cent of women said sex was an important component of their relationship with their partner. Quite impressively, 74 per cent of the sexually active men and 70 per cent of the sexually active women reported being as satisfied or more satisfied with their sexual lives than when they were in their 40s.[59] Don't you love it when science dispels stereotypes?

Another study conducted in 2006 looked at women aged 52–90 who remarried after the age of 50.[60] Most said they'd experienced strong sexual chemistry with their later-life husbands. It was suggested that 'sexual novelty' contributed to the sexual chemistry initially experienced by the women. However, *all* of the women interviewed said sexual intercourse was not a priority in their remarriage relationships, regardless of the presence or absence of health problems or other barriers to maintaining an active sexual life. Sexual intercourse was less important than it had been when the women were younger, while other ways of expressing love and affection, namely companionship, hugging, cuddling, and kissing, were more valued. Indeed, companionship is an especially potent redirected form of eros. Non-genital pleasures—found in shared activities, affection, acts of kindness, and a plethora of other delights—strengthen the bond between couples and make up for loss of desire. After all, who wants to have sex when you can watch cop shows together with a nice cup of tea?

An active sex life, it has been suggested, can increase the human life span. In the UK, a government health adviser went so far as to officially promote the advantages of sex to the elderly. Ian Philp stated that regular sex and plenty of money in the bank are the key to a long and healthy life.[61] Goodness, if it were only so easy.

Menopause and libido

The extent to which menopause transition is associated with decreased sexual functioning versus ageing *per se* is an area of hot academic debate.[62] Although many studies indicate that sexual functioning declines, so far it's too hard to figure out definitively what part of this is related to menopause, ageing or other variables.[63]

Some researchers have found that during the menopausal transition, women experience changes in their sexual response and a significant increase in sexual problems.[64] A 2009 study headed by Nancy Avis (looking at 3302 women across America) found that pain during sexual intercourse *increases* and sexual desire *decreases* over the menopausal transition, although sexual frequency doesn't change much.[65] In part, this mirrored the Melbourne Women's Midlife Health Project findings, which saw greater declines in sexual function (decreases in desire, arousal, orgasm, frequency of sexual activities, and increasing vaginal dryness/dyspareunia) as women transitioned from premenopause to postmenopause.[66] The Penn Ovarian Aging study in the US also found an increase of overall sexual 'dysfunction' with advanced menopausal status, with postmenopausal women being 2.3 times more likely to experience sexual 'dysfunction' compared with premenopausal women.[67] However, later analysis of findings from the Melbourne study showed that previous sexual function and relationship factors affected libido and sexual responsiveness more than oestradiol level.[68]

Looking at why women have decreased libido in their late reproductive years, Clarisa Gracia and her colleagues conducted a study of 326 women over four years based on hormone assays and questionnaires. Vaginal dryness, depression and children living at home negatively affected sex drive. Women whose testosterone levels fluctuated more during the study were more likely to report low libido. This indicates that *variations* in hormones, as distinct from their absolute levels, relate to specific menopausal symptoms.[69] While some studies indicate that a decline in oestrogen or androgen levels is linked to sexual dysfunction during the menopausal transition, findings are contradictory and inconclusive.[70] It is not clear why sexual function declines during the menopausal transition; ultimately the relationship between hormonal changes and sexuality during this time is elusive.[71]

Lorraine Dennerstein and Janet Guthrie (2008) conducted an eleven-year study of Australian menopausal women's sexuality.[72] (Note, lead researcher Lorraine Dennerstein has received grant money, consulting fees and the reimbursement of travel expenses for attending expert panels for a number of leading drug companies.)

Compared with the first year, at the eleventh year of follow-up, there was *a significant decline in all areas of sexual function and relationship factors studied*: 81 per cent of participants had low sexual function. Of these, however, only one in five were sexually distressed. Combining the results for low sexual function and sexual distress produced a female sexual dysfunction prevalence estimate of 17 per cent for Australian women aged 56–67.

Yet, although the majority of women in their fifties and sixties had low levels of sexual function, hardly any of them were worried about it, leading the authors to state that distress about low sexual function generally decreases with age. As I've suggested throughout, this indicates that many women stop seeing their sexuality through the limited lens of traditional heterosexist norms. Instead women often find a new sensuality in many varied things, like socialising, writing, gardening, taking care of grandchildren, companionship with their partner, friendship, religion, reflection or indeed sexual activities. They welcome a more diffuse sexuality, one not focused on the genitals or necessarily a partner, but on their own place and enjoyments in the world. Often, declining desire simply reflects a shift in women's priorities.

As for those women who did experience distress over their sexual problems, they were more likely to have more negative feelings for their partner, more reports of partners having problems with sexual performance, higher levels of depression and lower overall wellbeing. Surprise—their bad moods also manifested under the sheets. In terms of Hormone Replacement Therapy (HRT), the authors found that women on hormone treatments had a higher total sex score, greater responsiveness and higher frequency of sexual activities. Those with partners reported that their partners had fewer performance problems and that they had significantly greater positive feelings for their partners than postmenopausal women not using HRT.

In a 2006 study, Dennerstein, Grziottin, plus Proctor & Gamble employees Koochaki and Barton explored rates of HSDD among 2467 menopausal women aged 20 to 70 years in France, Germany, Italy and the UK.[73] It turned out that a greater proportion of surgically menopausal women had low sexual desire compared with premenopausal or naturally menopausal women. Low sexual desire usually meant sexual arousal, orgasm and sexual pleasure were low too. In terms of numbers, among premenopausal women 20 to 49 years of age the prevalence of HSDD was 7 per cent, and 16 per cent for surgically menopausal women. The prevalence of HSDD among women aged 50 to 70 was 9 per cent for naturally menopausal women and 12 per cent for surgically menopausal women. Results from these and other studies have led to the widely held view that removal of the ovaries reduces desire.

Menopause can be challenging, as women often experience a wide variety of conditions that may cause changes in their sexual function. A woman's concept of herself as a sexual being also often shifts during menopause. Mood swings, hot flushes and vaginal dryness—it's not hard to understand why so many menopausal women lose touch with their libido. Some find they don't think about sex like they used to, others want to have sex but don't enjoy it enough to justify the effort, while others again take it upon themselves to seduce.

Self-image

Whatever our age, self-image is often a major factor in a woman's sex drive. If we are uncomfortable with the way our body has changed during menopause, we may be less inclined to share physical intimacy. Appearance issues in relation to weight gain, incontinence and changes in our skin and breasts can affect the way we feel about our sexuality.

Inversely, some menopausal women feel like they've spent *too much* of their life being self-conscious about their body and their sexuality. They are able to radically refocus their energies, and by doing so find sex newly pleasurable. Many also enjoy a new array of nonsensual pursuits.

Partner issues

Another important aspect of ageing and libido is the impact of a partner's sexual ailments. Often the male partner initiates sexual activity but with ageing this may decrease owing to issues associated erectile dysfunction, a major source of poor body image and resulting low desire for men. Although Viagra has aided many men in the war against the flaccid penis, it has also caused a serious shift in many couples' sexual equilibrium. Just as women first had to adjust to the sexual equilibrium of abstinence, now they must accommodate another change. Sheryl Kingsberg writes: 'Not only do older people require a longer adjustment period to make the necessary accompanying cognitive shift, but older women definitely need time for their bodies to readjust to a partnered sexual life.'[74] However, she adds, give a man a reliable erection and he usually wants to use it. 'Unfortunately, if he and his partner have not had intercourse for a long time, her aging vagina has likely narrowed and atrophied and will not immediately accommodate a penis without risking pain and/or injury.'[75]

Not being a lesbian

Yep. Sociologist Julie Winterich's research on heterosexual and lesbian women's experience of menopause found that they had differing attitudes to sexual issues such as vaginal dryness and changes in libido.[76] Lesbian participants with sexual problems, for instance, went about their business in a very civilised way. They tended to engage in open dialogue with their partners about their sexual needs and showed greater willingness to adapt their sexual activities. And they used a broader definition of 'sex' than their heterosexual participants, who, reflecting the dominant culture, focused more on the genitals and orgasm. Winterich found that heterosexual women had difficulty discussing their sexual preferences with their husbands, dealing with their husbands' complaints about vaginal dryness, and faking orgasms. Of course, many lebsian couples also experience disparity in sexual wellbeing.

> Diane, 57, lives in Queensland, part-time job in retail, married for 30 years, mother of three
>
> **Could you tell me about your experiences with menopause?**
>
> I went through menopause, finished it four years ago. I suffered from very bad depression, and had a few episodes when I was around 50. It pushed me into a very black hole. I went into counselling for 12 months and was on antidepressants for four years. I weaned myself off those last year, which was very difficult. This depression was related to the hormonal changes going on.
>
> **What other menopause symptoms have you had?**
>
> I haven't had the full-blown night sweats, but I have had a few 'power surges', hot flushes. Only a dozen or so. I'm not very keen on any chemical balancing. I don't particularly believe in HRT [hormone replacement therapy], or anything of that nature.
>
> **Do you think your depression was solely related to menopause?**
>
> I think so. The only other time I had it really bad was between the age of 12 and 16. Which again is related to a hormonal—what would you call it—*imbalance* [she laughs].

Did your concept of your self change during menopause?

I think I'm a lot more confident and I know myself better than before, but it's hard to know whether that's age or menopause.

Was menopause a time of consolidation or liberation from old roles?

There's none of the false bullshit anymore. You can be comfortable in your skin. You don't have to be Miss Perfect, which is important especially for my generation—to look as young as you can, be everything, blah, blah, blah. I don't think it's as big of an issue for me.

Menopause often seems to be associated with loss—loss of youth, beauty and reproductive abilities. Does it feel like that?

Yes, I would say that. It only hit me now that I'm ... old. I put on weight, probably about 10 kilos, around the middle. I have dryness everywhere, dry skin, but I've always had dry skin. And sexual lubrication has disappeared now. My husband now has to always to use a lubricant, otherwise it's painful.

Does lubrication disturb the mood?

Yes, absolutely. I've got no libido now.

And you think this is solely related to menopause and hormones?

Yes.

Was it a gradual shift, this loss of desire?

Yes, a gradual decrease over five years.

So you've been married for 30 years, and for 25 years, until you started going through menopause, your libido was pretty steady, and now it's disappeared?

It was steady in the normal way—we all have ups and downs, and what happens when you have children—but yes. I think it's all related to lubrication, I really do. It's such an issue to go and get cream, no spontaneity. I can't be bothered.

How is your husband coping with your drop in desire?

He's coping okay with that. Of course he's older now . . . Maybe it's nature's way with coping with the female drop in libido. I do think men have the same thing.

Have you found new sensual pleasures?

My partner and I have become a lot closer because we're doing a lot more together than when we were working full time. Probably more friendship.

From my reading it seems like during our reproductive years we are very desire-focused, but as we get older that can change . . .

When you do have sex it's more . . . it's not panting . . . it's more familiar, relaxed. It's for a different reason, more companionable, not the highly sexed urges of when you were younger. You get

> into a rhythm with life; the more so, the longer you are with a partner. You try things, go through stages, looks, the way that you dress, the way you perceive yourself and how others perceive you. You don't put so much pressure on yourself, you give yourself more permission to relax. You can't fight it, no matter how much surgery or Botox you have.

Despite the different factors that can stand in the way of feeling sexy, many women undergoing menopause or who are post-menopause are content with their new lowered sex drive and do not wish to seek treatment of any sort. The departure of sex is experienced as essentially liberating, as a time to focus their energy on other things. Others experience a resurgence of desire in later life; the power they have as mature women is translated to sexual power.

Melbourne herbalist and natural fertility management author Wendy Dumaresq puts it this way:

I have found quite a few women to have a different attitude about their sexuality than when they were younger. They are more open in their relationship about their needs, they are less concerned about saying 'no' and care less about what others think about them on the whole, which can be very empowering. Quite a few women I know have stated that they are 'just not interested in sex or sexuality anymore—that they have more important things to think about'. Also very liberating I think! I feel that it is a natural transition in a woman's life sometimes at this age and stage to have less emphasis on sexuality and more on 'soul'-centred living.[77]

When it comes to reclaiming sexual desire in the context of ageing, one often overlooked option is expanding or changing sexual repertoire. Many of us have pretty narrow lines about what 'sex' is. Let us consider redefining 'normal' sexual behaviour and reconceptualising intercourse as the main event. Lesbians do. This is a particularly good idea for couples experiencing genital atrophy or erectile dysfunction. And a tip: make love in the morning, when couples, old and young alike, have more energy.

The use of lubricants can make intercourse less painful and more enjoyable for older women, although they can admittedly disrupt spontaneity and flow. Creams that contain oestrogen can also be applied to the vagina to restore its walls to a healthier state and increase the ability to produce vaginal mucus. Hormone replacement therapy may not chemically boost libido, but it may help reduce other symptoms that may be complicating a woman's sex life (see Chapter 9).

It is possible for us to actively resist and challenge the notion that to age is to lose our sexual vitality. Health providing, what these later years grant us is time—free time, which may be the most precious aphrodisiac of all. Our libido no longer needs to be confined to a reproductive, one-partner, hegemonic terrain, but can open up, become diffuse, and mean many varied things.

It is up to us to discover pleasure, to create our own *jouissance*. It is up to us to accept our ageing body—plumper, drier, slower, or what have you—and dabble in what makes life divine. Be it water aerobics, be it family, be it sex.

After all, as the Guatemalan proverb goes, 'Everyone is the age of their heart.' Even if we have a dry vagina.

9

Sex drugs

Somewhere in Continental Europe. Two women in their 30s are touching up their make-up in a *chi chi* restaurant bathroom. The brunette takes a little spray bottle out of her handbag, pulls up her A-line skirt and sprays her inner thigh. The other woman raises her eyebrow and the brunette smiles, explaining, 'I'm on a date. It's *Eros Breeze* . . .'

Given recent technological advances, the increase of understanding in neurobiology, and our sex-fuelled culture, it's difficult to even imagine the potential future of post-modern libidos. Will it be a world of teledildonics, where we use computers to control sex toys over long distances? Will treatments be available to stop physical ageing, to keep our bodies young and beautiful and sexually appealing? And will a chemical concoction crack the 'crisis' in women's sexuality and make us want to fuck even after a long day's work?

At present, there are a number of drug options for women experiencing sexual problems. Besides ecstasy. But almost all of the drugs targeting female libido aren't on sale at a pharmacy. Many desire enhancers are currently being trialled—for the second or third time—while most have been flat-out rejected by regulators such as the Australian TGA (Therapeutic Goods Administration) and the FDA (the American Food and Drug Administration) because they haven't been considered safe or effective enough for public consumption. In other words, we're close, but no cigar.

Upon deeper investigation, though, it is clear that many doctors prescribe sex drugs 'off label', without knowing their true effectiveness or long-term health effects. 'Off label' refers to the use of a legally available drug for an unapproved purpose. Off-label use is extremely common. A 2001 study showed that 21 per cent of total prescriptions in the US were off-label, and that approximately 73 per cent of all off-label use had little or no scientific support.[1] While it is legal and common for physicians to prescribe off-label drugs in most countries, it is illegal for pharmaceutical companies to directly promote drugs for off-label use. But this is poorly policed, and companies take advantage of grey areas in legislation and enforcement. In the US between 2003 and 2008, federal prosecutors and state attorneys-general brought more than a dozen cases against drug makers for off-label marketing and won more than $6 billion in criminal and civil settlements.[2]

It is almost certain, however, that a sexual cure-all is on its way to a pharmacy near you. Not usually a gambling woman, I have a number of reasons to be confident in saying so. First off, given the success of Viagra, finding its female equivalent is an obvious goal. Second, the number of drug-company-backed scientists in hot pursuit of a sexual fortifier for women is similar to the backing received for walking on the moon—lots of hard science, lots of hard cash. Third, a whole new discipline has been created called 'sexual medicine'. Fourth, the sophisticated state of current brain research promises discoveries about where lust and desire are located in the human brain and how to amplify them. This will inform the creation of a sexual elixir that changes not only our body's reaction to stimuli, but how we think about that reaction. It's likely that research on hormones and blood flow will also become more compelling. Fifth, marital sex has become the bedrock of measuring marital happiness, with divorce or adultery a common response to lack of sexual satisfaction. Sixth, our sexuality is becoming increasingly medicalised, treated as though it were a medical condition requiring intervention. Too many people believe the hype that a low libido is a dysfunction. Dysfunctions, of course, require drugs, and there is little doubt that the future will bring a cornucopia of pharmaceutical potions. After all, seventh reason, we are already doped up. We are already used to taking drugs that tamper with our hormones and central nervous system. We are already used to a body supplemented by the artificial. From designer foods to designer dogs to designer babies to designer brains to designer Viagra penises, we left nature a long time ago. Sex drugs are part of our common landscape: the contraceptive pill and hormone replacement therapy (HRT) are now ordinary aids in our complicated modern life, and not seen as the strange and miraculous chemical compounds that they are.

As a culture, we are becoming increasingly medicated. Add too the devastating effects of antidepressants on libido, and the alarming number of people on antidepressants, and there is cause for global concern. Our bodies are unarguably less aligned with nature than at any other time in human history. Where once we were pioneers of land and sea, now we are pioneers of consumption, used to absorbing substances that alter our normal bodily function, be they Valium, Zoloft, or the plethora of pills we are prescribed for illness and to fight off the ravages of ageing.

Like postmodern brothels, the pharmaceutical companies produce increasingly more sophisticated and alluring drugs. Nootropics, for example, aka 'smart drugs', work to improve cognitive abilities, such as memory, concentration, thought, mood and learning. Some nootropics are now being used to help people regain brain functioning lost during ageing, and to treat diseases such as Alzheimer's.

New markets are also being found for existing drugs. Beta blockers, originally prescribed for conditions such as angina and hypertension, are commonly used by musicians and actors to reduce stage fright. Ritalin, the drug used to treat ADHD, is being taken by exam-cramming uni students to improve concentration during all-nighters.

And so medicine has replaced magic, and doctors and lab researchers have replaced the shamans and herbalists of yesteryear. We can turn a man into a woman, stop female fertility, alter melancholy, and reverse hormonal changes associated with menopause so that women feel 35 again.

Well, then, what can the enterprise of medicine do for our tired, lagging libidos?

Female sexual ennui is a problem pharmaceutical companies believe they are in the best position to solve. Next we

Sex drugs: female libido

Product	Company	General target	Primarily for?	What is it?	Available?
Flibanserin	Boehringer Ingelheim	Central nervous system	HSDD	A tablet, originally designed as an antidepressant. Reduces serotonin levels, thereby reduces signals from the brain that inhibit desire.	Not approved in Australia or the US. Rejected by the FDA in June 2010 because it only marginally increased frequency of sex and raised safety concerns (dizziness, fainting, insomnia, fatigue). Boehringer Ingelheim have put research on hold.
Bupropion	GlaxoSmithKline	Central nervous system	HSDD, SAD	Sold as an antidepressant and smoking cessation aid, but shows promise as a sex agent and is used off-label for sexual dysfunction. Binds to dopamine receptors, increasing sexual responsiveness. One of the few antidepressants to not cause sexual dysfunction. Side effects: skin reactions, psychiatric disturbances, problems involving the nervous system and gastrointestinal tract.	Approved by the FDA as an antidepressant in 1985; reintroduced in 1989 after original dose was found to cause seizures. Approved in 1997 in the US as a smoking cessation aid and also approved in Australia for this purpose. Off-label use for HSDD.
Bremelanotide (previously PT-141)	Palatin Technologies	Central nervous system	HSDD, SAD	Synthetic a-melanocortin-stimulating drug. Affects the central nervous system, triggering increased sexual desire and genital arousal. Experimental subcutaneous (under skin) delivery.	Impending phase II trial discussions with FDA. Previous trials of PT-141 (nasal delivery) were stopped when the FDA rejected the drug for risk of increased blood pressure.

Product	Company	General target	Primarily for?	What is it?	Available?
Oestradiol (Vagifem, Ovestin, Estraderm)	Upjohn, Novartis, Schering-Plough	Hormonal system	SAD (HRT)	The primary oestrogen. Vaginal tablet, cream, pessary or patch to improve vaginal dryness and elasticity.	Yes, widely available.
Methyltestosterone with esterified oestrogens (Estratest)	Solvay	Hormonal system	HSDD, SAD	Form of HRT that combines methyltestosterone and esterfied oestrogens in one pill. Methltestosterone is a synthetic testosterone derivative.	Solvay discontinued production of Estratest in 2009 and many others followed suit. Not FDA approved due to safety concerns and unproven efficacy. Prescribed off-label in US. Not approved by TGA or available in Australia.
Premarin with methyl-testosterone	Wyeth	Hormonal system	HSDD, arousal disorder (+ HRT)	Taken orally. Premarin is a compound drug of synthetic oestrogens. Methyl-testosterone is a synthetic testosterone derivative.	Methyl-testosterone with oestrogen is not approved by the FDA or TGA for any medical use. Doctors in the US prescribe off-label.
Testosterone (Intrinsa)	Procter & Gamble	Hormonal system	HSDD	A 300 µg testosterone patch, applied twice weekly to the abdomen. For surgically menopausal women with HSDD (under 60 only).	Rejected by the FDA in 2004 due to concerns about its long-term safety. Not approved or available in the US, Canada, Asia or Australia. Available in Europe since 2006 only for surgically menopausal women as a last resort. Undergoing trials in Australia.
Testosterone (LibiGel)	BioSante Pharmaceuticals	Hormonal system	HSDD	Testosterone gel, applied to the upper arm.	BioSante anticipate new drug application in 2012. Unlikely to be approved in the next few years.

Product	Company	General target	Primarily for?	What is it?	Available?
Testosterone (AndroFeme)	Lawley Pharmaceuticals	Hormonal system	HSDD	1 per cent testosterone cream. Applied once daily to the inner arms or upper outer thighs.	Available only in Western Australia, but can be bought online.
Testosterone (Luramist, Testosterone, MDTS)	Acrux	Hormonal system	HSDD	Metered dose testosterone spray (MDTS)	Acrux was squabbling with its former licensee Vivus during 2009 over delays to commencement of phase 3 trials, before forcefully regaining the US rights. Acrux were seeking a partner to develop Luramist in 2010 however have been very quiet since 2011.
Prasterone (DHEA) (Prestara)	Generic and Genelabs Technologies	Hormonal system	HSDD, SAD	DHEA (dehydroepiandrosterone) is a precursor to testosterone and oestrogen, recent research has shown no effect.	Off-label use (often prescribed for lupus). Can be bought over the counter in the US and by prescription in Canada. Not approved in Australia.
Tibolone (Livial)	Organon	Hormonal system	HSDD, SAD (HRT)	Synthetic hormone, sold as a tablet. Said to improve vaginal dryness and overall sexual function. Has oestrogenic effects, activates androgen receptors and increases circulating free testosterone. Mainly used for HRT in postmenopausal women. Possible increased risk of ischaemic stroke in women over 60.	Not approved in the US. Available in the UK, other parts of Europe and Australia.

Product	Company	General target	Primarily for?	What is it?	Available?
Sildenafil (Viagra)	Pfizer Lilly	Peripheral vaginal/clitoral blood flow	SAD	Tablet. Relaxes vascular smooth muscles and widens blood vessels, enhancing circulation.	Off-label use for women.
NMI-870	NitroMed	Peripheral vaginal/clitoral blood flow	SAD	Nitric oxide (NO)-enhanced compound of the alpha-2 blocker yohimbine. Purported to cause an increase in localised nitric oxide, enhancing circulation and arousal.	Not yet. Phase II clinical trials demonstrated increased vaginal blood flow in postmenopausal women with SAD.
L-arginine amino acid (ArginMax)	Daily Wellness Company	Peripheral vaginal/clitoral blood flow	SAD	Purported to provide L-arginine, a building block for nitric oxide, and increase nitric oxide production, leading to enhanced blood circulation and arousal.	Sold in Australia as a cosmetic and varous other products are sourced from overseas via internet. 2002 application to TGA to use it in listable medicines as long as not used on the vagina or rectum (irritation risk). An earlier application for oral ingestion was rejected due to evidence that it stimulated breast tumours.
Alprostadil (prostaglandin E1) (Femprox)	Apricus Biosciences	Peripheral vaginal/clitoral blood flow	SAD	Prostaglandin E1 cream is claimed to increase blood flow to the genitals by relaxing vascular smooth muscles.	Femprox: Apricus Bio claims to have completed nine clinical studies, including one phase II study in the US and a proof-of-concept phase II–III study in China.

FDA: Food and Drug Administration (USA)
HRT: hormone replacement therapy
HSDD: hypoactive sexual desire disorder
SAD: sexual arousal disorder
TGA: Therapeutic Goods Administration

will look at some of the drugs designed to resurrect female desire. These are either available at the pharmacy, under trial, steadily being worked upon in the race to develop—and patent—the perfect concoction or abandoned . . . for now. As we will see, many drugs experience rebirth, and are used in different ways, for different purposes, by different companies. These drugs described in the chapter are a mixed bag in terms of safety and efficacy. But trust me, one of them, or a close relative, will come out on top, and get *us* on top.

Sex drugs—blood flow
Viagra, Cialis, Levitra

In the mid-1990s, researchers at Pfizer were testing an experimental drug for angina and made an interesting discovery . . . their male subjects were experiencing persistent hard-ons. Flash forward to 1998 and Viagra (sildenafil) hits the market, changing the play of sex forever. Originally meant to redeem a medical problem, it became *the* lifestyle drug. Viagra, however, wasn't an overnight success. It took several years for both the medical establishment and patients to become comfortable with it, and millions of marketing dollars to turn it into a household name with blockbuster sales.[3]

Since Viagra's entrance to the scene, followed by its groupies Cialis (tadalafil) and Levitra (vardenafil), drug makers have been searching for a female equivalent. Viagra was the first in a class of drugs known as phosphodiesterase 5 (PDE5) inhibitors, which increase blood flow to the genitals by raising levels of nitric oxide, which encourages relaxation and dilation of blood vessels. Given erectile dysfunction is considered more of a physical problem than an emotional one, Viagra works well for many men.

Limited research has shown that women who take Viagra experience increased blood flow to the vagina and clitoris.[4] Some research has indicated that Viagra may reduce the adverse side effect of sexual dysfunction in women taking SSRI antidepressants.[5] However, many of these studies were conducted with small sample sizes, or used inappropriate statistical tests or dubious non-validated assessment tools.[6] Interestingly the same names often appear as authors of these studies, most notably the Berman sisters—Laura and Jennifer, who were named 'the face of FSD' in the documentary movie *Orgasm, Inc.*. The Bermans' have become widely criticised for their close ties with Pfizer, who paid for the studies they developed and conducted on Viagra's effects on women.[7] When asked by *Time* magazine about her portrayal in *Orgasm Inc.*, Laura said 'I've never felt an ounce of pressure to create specific results or frame things in a certain way', and 'I really see the pharmaceutical companies as an ally'.[8]

In a 2008 paper, researchers Susan Davis and Esme Nijland write that the Viagra studies of the Bermans' and Basson[9] suggest that 'this therapy may be useful for some women with genital arousal disorder rather than the larger group of women with low desire and subjective arousal'. They conclude that 'large studies of PDE5 inhibitors in the general population have been disappointing'.[10]

So although Viagra may turn women on physically (getting us wet), it doesn't turn us on mentally. Physical arousal doesn't necessarily translate into wanting sex.

Sex drugs: hormone supplementation

A number of factors affect the balance of hormone levels over our lifetime. Some are age related, such as the relatively sudden changes in oestrogen levels that occur with the onset of menopause, as well as the slower and less perceptible decline in women's androgen levels from our 30s onwards. (Androgens are hormones that create secondary male sex characteristics such as facial or body hair, thicker skin, increased muscle mass and deeper voice. The leading man of androgens is testosterone.)

Other hormonal changes may occur as a result of disease or surgery. These include hypopituitarism, hypogonadism, polycystic ovarian syndrome, and the removal of ovaries and other reproductive organs. Some hormonal changes arise from taking the oral contraceptive pill. Hormone replacement therapy also has a significant effect on our hormones.

We now turn our attention to the pharmaceutical treatments currently being used to alter hormone levels in the body, and then some leading edge hormone research.

Hormone replacement therapy (HRT)

The contraceptive pill is not the only drug relating to our sexuality that's become an international habit. Women disturbed by the naturally ageing body can purchase seemingly magical drugs to alter their hormonal make-up. Hormone replacement therapy (HRT) involves supplementing the body's natural hormones. It is commonly used for menopause and, not so commonly, for transgender therapy and androgen therapy in men and women. Younger women with premature ovarian failure or surgical menopause may also use HRT until the age when natural menopause would likely occur.

HRT has been controversial, with medical professionals flip-flopping over its risks and benefits for the past five decades, from thinking it's gold, to poison, and back again.

HRT aims to treat the discomfort caused by diminished circulating hormones in surgically menopausal, perimeno-pausal and, to a lesser extent, postmenopausal women. It increases levels of the hormones the ovaries have stopped producing, mainly oestrogen and progesterone. Oestrogen and progesterone are prescribed in a variety of combinations, and sometimes testosterone is also added in the hope of increasing sex drive, restoring energy levels and preventing osteoporosis.

HRT is often given for short-term relief from menopausal symptoms such as hot flushes, irregular menstruation, night sweats, vaginal dryness and urinary symptoms. Studies comparing HRT with a placebo show strong evidence that HRT is effective for such symptoms.[11]

HRT can be delivered by way of patches, tablets, creams, troches, IUDs, vaginal rings, gels or, more rarely, by injection.

Evidence shows that HRT may improve some aspects of sexual function, such as a reduction in dryness; oestrogen therapy can also have a positive effect on brain function and mood factors that affect sexual response.[12] That said, some research also suggests that HRT has a negative impact on libido (as well as depressive effects). A 1997 study found that an increase in oestrogen arising from oestrogen-containing pills inhibits androgen production in the ovaries.[13] Other researchers found oestrogen therapy binds up free testosterone, hence lowering its availability, and possibly leading to low sexual desire.[14] (More on androgen deficiency a little later on.)

HRT is plagued by controversy. In the 1960s bestseller *Feminine Forever*,[15] Robert Wilson framed menopause as an oestrogen-deficiency disease, preaching that all peri-menopausal women should take oestrogen for the remainder of their lives rather than face the inevitable 'living decay'. Women listened. This idea of preserving youth and beauty through HRT has been promoted more recently by pharmaceutical companies in advertisements that 'convey the message that oestrogens are a cure-all for the anxious, wrinkled, sexually frustrated older woman who has to compete in this era of cocktail parties, sexual freedom and errant husbands'.[16]

Then, in the 1970s, oestrogen replacement therapy was found to increase the risk of endometrial cancer. Talk about bad publicity. So doctors stopped prescribing HRT. Jump ahead a few years, and new studies showed some health benefits if oestrogen was combined with progesterone. Throughout the 1980s and 1990s, many doctors went back to prescribing HRT, telling their patients it would help prevent heart disease. Nevertheless, HRT was now recognised as having both positive and negative effects.

Attitudes towards HRT changed again in 2002 when the US National Institutes of Health announced that women receiving a form of HRT called Prempro (conjugated equine oestrogens and a progestin) had a larger incidence of breast cancer, heart attacks and strokes. As a result of these findings the *Journal of the American Medical Association* recommended that women with natural (rather than surgical) menopause should take the lowest feasible dose of HRT for the shortest possible time to minimise risks.[17] Millions of women immediately went off HRT. Cold turkey.

The Women's Health Initiative (WHI) Estrogen-Alone Trial, conducted from 1993 to 1998, evaluated the effects of conjugated equine oestrogens on the incidence of chronic disease among postmenopausal women (age 50 to 79) who had had a hysterectomy. The trial was stopped a year early because of an increased risk of stroke. At the time it was concluded that this treatment should not be recommended to prevent chronic disease in postmenopausal women.[18] However, because treatment effects differed by age, follow up was required. In the WHI follow-up study though 2009, it was found that younger women (age 50 to 59) receiving conjugated equine oestrogens had slightly lower risk of coronary heart disease and other diseases. Also, oestrogen use was not associated with excess risk for stroke or other problems such as deep-vein thrombosis, hip fracture and colorectal cancer.[19] Today it is understood that oestrogen-alone therapy is safe for as long as six years for young menopausal women (age 50 to 59) who have had a hysterectomy.

As for oestrogen plus progestin (E+P), the WHI trial found that Prempro—the combination of conjugated equine oestrogens and medroxyprogesterone—was associated with coronary heart disease and breast cancer.[20] The trial was stopped after the coronary heart disease and breast cancer risks were found to exceed the benefits. For every 10,000 women taking E+P, 41 women each year will develop breast cancer, as compared to 33 women per year who would develop breast cancer while taking a placebo. Also, the breast cancers that developed in women taking E+P were larger and more advanced; about 25 per cent had spread to lymph nodes or elsewhere in the body, compared to 16 per cent in women taking a placebo.[21]

There have also been cases of accidental exposure to HRT. An increasing number of hormone gels, creams and sprays are associated with cases in which users unwittingly exposed children and pets to HRT hormones. For instance, in 2010, Acrux, the Australian manufacturer of Evamist (an oestrogen spray for relief of menopause symptoms) warned women not to use their product in front of children or pets. This warning was issued after its American arm reported at least 10 cases of exposure to pets and children, resulting in children aged three to five displaying symptoms of early puberty, including enlarged breasts and nipple soreness.[22] Evamist was approved in the US in 2007, but is yet to be approved by Australia's Therapeutic Goods Administration.

Designer hormones

Although HRT usually comprises synthetic one-size-fits-all drug combinations such as Premarin, Prempro, and Provera, women in the US are increasingly opting for bioidentical hormone replacement therapy (HRT), with celebrities such as Oprah Winfrey, actress Suzanne Somers and Robin McGraw, the wife of talk-show host Dr Phil, fronting the trend.

Using an individualised approach, blood tests are taken to determine the woman's hormone levels. (Other tests—on urine, saliva, hair follicles—can also be conducted.) Then a calculated dosage of bioidentical oestrogens, progesterone, pregnenalone, testosterone and/or DHEA is prescribed and prepared, usually at a compounding pharmacy. The patient is then monitored through regular follow-up hormone tests to ensure symptom relief is maintained at the lowest possible dosage.

Celebrities are endorsing bioidenticals as the new fountain of youth.

Suzanne Somers' 2004 book *The Sexy Years: Discover the Hormone Connection—The secret to fabulous sex, great health, and vitality, for women and men* touts the benefits of bioidenticals as 'natural hormones'.[23] Robin McGraw appeared on Oprah alongside menopause guru, Dr Christiane Northrup in 2010, and also sang the praises of bioidentical hormones. Her 2008 book *What's Age Got To Do With It?* details her personal journey to hormone balance. So there's another item to add to the list: work–life balance, emotional balance, and now, hormonal balance. But unlike the others, you can *buy* this type of harmony.

Fans of bioidenticals extol the use of hormones not just to combat menopause, but as lifestyle drugs to minimise health risks, improve quality of life (for now at least—forget any long-term consequences) and to ensure that, like Peter Pan, we never grow old. It is believed that bioidenticals can make women feel young again and restore their hormone levels back to those of a 30-year-old. The ethos is clear: take charge of your health and buy back your youth, your soft skin, your wet vagina, your sex drive.

Amazingly, Robin McGraw has also got her hubby, Dr Phil, on these controversial drugs. She writes:

> . . . after everything I learned about my own body,
> I learned a few things about Philip's, too, and that's when
> I started *him* on supplements. He trusts my research and
> hard work so much that he takes whatever I suggest (and
> feels a lot better for it), and he even lets me drag him to
> have his blood drawn every once in a while.[24]

Holy smokes.

The answer to McGraw's quest to manage her hormones
came in the form of The Hall Health & Longevity Center in
California, and its founder Dr Prudence Hall, whose motto
is, 'Anyone who has a low hormone should have it replaced.'[25]

Hormone replacement, then, is for everybody. In fact, for
optimal living, McGraw says we should all start monitoring
our hormones in our . . . twenties! That way, she adds, by
the time menopause comes along, we probably won't have
any symptoms at all. Apparently premenstrual syndrome,
irregular or heavy periods, weight gain or exhaustion can
all indicate hormone imbalance or thyroid problems—and
as McGraw says, 'A little fatigue or weight gain here or
irritability or bloating there makes it [life] even harder, and it
doesn't have to be that way.'[26] She even took her 30-year-old
daughter-in-law to Dr Hall to get her hormones managed.

The American bioidentical advocate Christiane Northrup
has found a clever way of undermining conventional HRT,
specifically Premarin.[27] In addition to focusing on its known
risks and side effects, she often repeats that Premarin is
synthetic, unnatural and made from horse urine.[27] She
implies that the one-size-fits-all approach of conventional
HRT means you are not in control, not treated as a unique

person. Northrup appears to be tapping into the fashionable preference for 'green and natural' products. But the fact that we already have a chemical in our body does not necessarily make it right or safe to add more.

With conventional HRT there are risks. The risk with bioidenticals is that we do not know the risks: no studies exist on their long-term effects. Also, when drugs are made up, or compounded, at a pharmacy, they are not necessarily approved in that form by the regulator, so buyers have to trust the pharmacy's quality-control standards. In 2008 the FDA warned seven American pharmacy operations that their claims about the safety and effectiveness of BHRT were unsupported by medical evidence and thus considered false and misleading. Northrup believes that transdermal (skin) patches are the most physiologically appropriate way to take hormones, but this presents an increased risk to children and others who may accidentally put on or come in contact with a patch. Assuming bioidenticals are safe is potentially dangerous, especially given the track record of standard HRT.

Moreover, as Dr Wulf Utian, head of the North American Menopause Society, states, 'There's no such thing as a natural hormone. They're all made in the lab, one way or another.'[28] He advises going with conventional drugs, which are approved by the regulator, and on the lowest possible hormone dose. But with a little digging you find that Utian has financial links to a number of pharmaceutical companies—so if you were feeling sceptical you might think the doctor had a reason or two to pitch conventional, *patentable* HRT.

Certainly Northrup believes much of the resistance to bioidentical hormones stems from the lack of incentive for pharmaceutical companies to produce something that cannot be patented. She also refers to the potential low price of bioidentical formulations: Dr Joel Hargrove's dropper-bottle approach (hormones dissolved in propylene glycol) can cost as little as $70 per year.[29]

Despite the known and unknown dangers of BHRT, it seems to be on a fast track to mainstream popularity. Perhaps one day there will be hormone servicers like ATMs that, with an instantaneous prick, measure our blood or saliva and pop out a little tube of perfectly concocted hormone cream to make us more 'us' and less old—and, for an extra fiver, give us a shot of antidepressant optimism spray.

Androgen therapy

There is a lot of fuss in the field of sexuality about testosterone. A number of medical practitioners, scientists and pharmaceutical companies believe that women's low libido can relate to low levels of androgens, including testosterone.

In women, androgen levels do not appear to fall suddenly with natural menopause as oestrogen levels do, but decline with increasing age—most likely owing to reduced production in the ovaries and lessened adrenal function. Total circulating and free (available) testosterone in women in their 40s is about half that in women in their 20s. Hence age-related androgen loss may occur in women in their late 30s and 40s.[30]

Other things that can lead to androgen loss include the use of oral contraceptives (the Pill) and oral oestrogens

(HRT), hypopituitarism, adrenal insufficiency, ovarian insufficiency, glucocorticoid therapy and oophorectomy (surgical removal of one or both ovaries, which makes testosterone levels fall by as much as half within 24 hours of surgery).[31]

Androgen deficiency is highly controversial and nebulously defined as, 'Complaints of a diminished sense of wellbeing, persistent unexplained fatigue, decreased sexual desire, sexual receptivity and pleasure by a woman who is oestrogen-replete and in whom no other significant contributing factors can be identified.'[32] Note there is no testosterone level specified, as a lower limit of 'normal' has not been established—and 'even within a so-called normal population there is a wide range of normality'.[33]

Some researchers believe female androgen deficiency can cause symptoms such as lethargy and loss of sexual interest. Others do not think there is a link between testosterone levels and low libido. Others again think the condition, if it exists at all, is too poorly understood to treat safely.

Testosterone replacement for men has been available since the 1930s, particularly for those suffering from hypogonadism (decreased functioning of the gonads), and men who have lost their testicular function to disease, cancer or other causes, giving rise to the medical term *andropause* and its pop culture counterpart, *manopause*. Androgen therapy has been shown to increase alertness, wellbeing and lean muscle mass, and enhance libido and the ability to achieve erection. For decades, men with low sex drives have been prescribed products containing large amounts of the hormone. However, it also has some adverse effects, such as increasing a man's red-blood-cell concentration (potentially leading to conditions such as heart attack and stroke). It has also been associated with sleep apnoea, acceleration of pre-existing prostate cancer and, in rare cases, liver toxicity.

There are several testosterone products for sale via patch, tablet, pill, cream, long-acting depot injection or the more recently developed buccal system (a patch applied to the upper gum). Apparently there has been a 500 per cent increase in prescription sales of testosterone products for men since 1993.[34] Also, much of what has worked for men is apparently being used on women, off-label. Physicians, lacking approved alternatives, have been giving female patients small doses of testosterone products in the hope of boosting desire without side effects. Fingers crossed.

Over the past decade, a number of studies have shown that testosterone may be important for women, especially in terms of staying fit and sexually active. Some studies show that testosterone therapy helps older women, restoring sex drive and sexual fantasies.

Most research has been performed in women who have undergone menopause or have had both ovaries removed (oophorectomy), or who have an underactive pituitary gland (hypopituitarism), because they are already low in important hormones. A number of these studies have been promising. Seemingly, if these women are given testosterone, their mood and sex drive increase. For example, a study in 2006 examined 51 premenopausal women with hypopituitarism. They received testosterone via a patch (300 μg/day) or placebo for 12 months. Afterwards, the free testosterone levels in those given the testosterone treatment had increased to the normal range, and their mood and sexual function also increased.[35]

A two-year study found that postmenopausal women receiving a combination of oestradiol and testosterone implants reported significantly greater scores for sexual activity, satisfaction, pleasure, and orgasm compared to women receiving oestradiol alone.[36] A 2008 study by Susan Davis and co-sponsored by Proctor & Gamble looked at the effects of testosterone on 814 surgically and naturally postmenopausal women diagnosed with HSDD. They found that a patch delivering 300 µg testosterone per day increased the number of self-reported sexually satisfying events per month when compared with placebo. The study also demonstrated significant improvement in desire, and sexual function and decrease personal distress in postmenopausal women.[37]

Health researchers Susan Davis and Esme Nijland suggest that women known to have loss of androgen production—surgically menopausal women, and those with adrenal insufficiency or hypopituitarism—merit consideration for testosterone treatment if they exhibit symptoms of sexual dysfunction.[38]

Several studies have found that a low testosterone level is *not* predictive of a diagnosis of low libido, and found no association between low sexual desire and function, and low levels of total testosterone, free testosterone or androstenedione.[39] In other words, having a low level of testosterone does not automatically mean a decline in sexual desire or function.

A 2005 study of 1423 Australian women aged 18 to 75 found that there is no single level of any hormone in the blood that separates women who report low sexual function from those who do not. However, women, particularly younger ones, who report low sexual function are more likely to have low levels of the hormone DHEAS.[40] DHEA and DHEAS are androgen precursors produced by the adrenal glands. They are converted in the body to testosterone and are the most abundant sex hormones in women.

There is no standard treatment for androgen deficiency in women. The worry is that most testosterone products, even low-dose ones, may contain too much testosterone for the female body to handle. No testosterone product has been government-approved to treat low libido in women in the US, Asia or South America, which has led to the off-label use of testosterone products commonly used by men, but in lower doses. Australian specialists familiar with this area generally recommend treatment with a low-dose 1 per cent testosterone cream (AndroFeme) or a low-dose subcutaneous pellet (off-label). AndroFeme is approved in Western Australia only.

Intrinsa, the skin patch in Susan Davis' aforementioned 2008 study, is approved in Europe. It is the first treatment for women with low libido to be available on prescription. After being rejected by the regulators in the US, Canada, Australia and Asia, Intrinsa gained approval in Europe in 2006. But not for everyone: it is available on prescription only for postmenopausal women with diagnosed sexual problems, or women who have premature menopause as a result of surgery. It was rejected by the FDA in 2004 *not* because it wasn't shown to work—in fact the panel voted 14 to 3 that the manufacturer's trials showed a meaningful improvement in desire and pleasure—but because data on safety were deemed insufficient.

The downside? Davis' 2008 study found that the improvement in sexual function was accompanied by 90 per cent more cases of increased hair growth than with placebo, three cases of clitoral enlargement, and two cases of breast cancer in the 267 participants receiving 300µg testosterone per day. Davis concluded that the long-term effects of testosterone, including effects on the breast, remain uncertain.[41]

Numerous other testosterone products are being tested on menopausal women. LibiGel, for example—a testosterone gel applied to the upper arm—is in phase III testing at the time of writing. Its manufacturer, BioSante Pharmaceuticals, is hopeful that Libigel will be the first product approved by the FDA for HSDD and anticipate submitting a new drug application in 2012.[42]

As for side effects, research is pretty limited. Testosterone implants and injections produce extremely high serum levels in women—often 10 times higher than normal levels, even when the hormones are administered in reduced doses. This can lead to side effects such as masculine physical characteristics, deepened voice, hair loss, acne, excessive hairiness and clitoral enlargement. Some of these side effects are irreversible.[43] A woman who chooses to have testosterone replacement therapy needs regular breast and pelvic examinations, mammography and evaluation for any abnormal bleeding by a doctor knowledgeable in this area.

As long-term safety data for testosterone therapy are lacking, some health experts advise that it should continue longer than six months only if there has been clear improvement in sexual function and satisfaction and absence of adverse effects.[44]

Another risk associated with testosterone treatment applied to the skin or in sprays is exposure to others, particularly children and pregnant women. A case was reported in 2010 of a four-year-old boy who was taken to a doctor after an unusual growth spurt and the development of a larger penis and pubic hair. Investigation revealed that for medical reasons his father was taking testosterone gel (50 mg daily) and that, during the past six months, the boy had been sleeping in his parents' bed.[45]

Another researcher describes three cases of partially irreversible virilisation of children whose fathers were using testosterone gel. One girl, aged two and a half, had been growing pubic hair for seven months, and had an enlarged (1.5 cm) clitoris and greasy hair; she also exhibited tomboyish behaviour and masturbated frequently. When gel exposure was stopped, it took two months for her clitoris to return to normal size and for masturbation to diminish; 14 months later she still exhibited tomboyish behaviour, and her bone age was two years older than her actual age.[46]

The FDA implemented label precautions in May 2008, but despite this eight new reports of child exposure were reported in the following six months. Most cases were attributed to patients failing to follow the label instructions and being unaware of the risk. I guess we're slow learners.

Premenopausal women and testosterone therapy

Numerous studies have shown that testosterone therapy has produced improvement in sex drive, arousal and frequency of sexual fantasies in women who are postmenopausal or have had their ovaries removed. However, we know little about the effects of androgen therapy in premenopausal women. There have been very few studies on testosterone therapy for premenopausal women.[47] Most studies of testosterone therapy actively *exclude* premenopausal women from participating owing to the risk of harm to the mother or foetus if pregnancy occurred during treatment.

The oral contraceptive pill, as we know[48] may affect androgen levels and decrease our sex drive. So first-line therapy for women experiencing low desire is to ditch the Pill and try a non-hormonal contraceptive such as the intrauterine device (IUD).

One of the American gurus of testosterone research, Jan Shifren, believes that healthy young women with regular menstrual cycles who are not receiving oral oestrogen therapy do not have a biological cause for low androgen concentrations and would not be likely to benefit from testosterone therapy. However, she says that 'there is interest in the role of androgen therapy for premenopausal women because many young women have sexual dysfunction'.[49]

And here lies our interest.

Australian researcher Susan Davis believes that because testosterone levels decline in women before menopause and do not appear to change across menopause, women in their late reproductive years are just as likely to have low testosterone levels as women in their early menopausal years.[50] Other researchers have proposed that women with low testosterone levels after menopause probably had low testosterone levels before menopause, and that sexual wellbeing before menopause is a good predictor of postmenopausal sexual wellbeing.[51]

Is testosterone therapy the answer to sexual dysfunction in premenopausal women?

A small trial headed by Rebecca Goldstat showed that premenopausal women treated with testosterone experienced significant improvements in sexual functioning and wellbeing compared to those given a placebo.[52]

In 2008, Susan Davis and her colleagues found that for premenopausal women aged 35 to 46 years with reduced libido and 'low' serum testosterone levels, a daily 90µL dose of testosterone spray increased the number of sexually satisfying episodes (SSEs) by approximately 0.8 per month. However the study lasted for only 16 weeks and the placebo effect was strong, with women on lower and higher doses reporting the same improvement as those receiving a placebo. No substantial relationships were found between free-testosterone levels and the number of SSEs during the study.[53]

Davis concludes that testosterone may prove to be a useful therapy for HSDD in premenopausal women, but says further studies are required to prove efficacy and safety.[54] Her work in this area continues. As of late 2011 Davis was recruiting premenopausal women aged 35 to 55 for a study to evaluate whether testosterone skin patches are effective in improving sexual interest, arousal and orgasm among women taking SSRI or SNRI antidepressants.[55]

Contemplating the widespread off-label use by women of testosterone products approved for men and the extensive prescription of testosterone products by doctors, Davis and her colleague Esme Nijland suggested that an uncontrolled clinical trial of the safety of testosterone is already happening in the community.[56]

Methyltestosterone

Methyltestosterone is a synthetic testosterone derivative. Estratest, a combination of methyltestosterone and esterified oestrogens, has been prescribed for decades to menopausal women with moderate to severe symptoms which did not improve with oestrogen alone. It is also administered to improve sexual desire and response. It is believed that methyltestosterone increases the bioavailable fraction of testosterone by decreasing SHBG levels (SHBG binds to testosterone). Rogiero Lobo and his colleagues found that its addition produced a greater improvement in sexual interest/desire than oestrogen alone.[57]

Since Estratest came onto the US market in 1964, over 36 million prescriptions have been filled (1965 to 2003). Estratest followed a number of other testosterone products in the US that were on the market before the FDA brought in its current stringent requirements for demonstrating safety and efficacy. Estratest was made available on the basis that it was equivalent to these earlier products. In 1981 the FDA prompted the manufacturer to apply for formal approval, however 25 years later the FDA had still not approved the application. In April 2003, the FDA concluded that the addition of testosterone to oestrogen products did not provide any greater relief for menopause symptoms. However, Estratest and equivalent generic brands remained on the market.[58]

In August 2003, a number of lawsuits were launched by people who claimed Solvay had used false and deceptive conduct in its marketing of Estratest. Solvay denied any wrongdoing.[59]

In August 2006 the National Women's Health Network petitioned the FDA to stop Solvay from marketing Estratest on the basis of unproven efficacy, known risks associated with oestrogen/testosterone products and other outstanding safety questions.[60] The FDA's rejection of Intrinsa in 2004 was a key lever in the argument against Estratest.[61]

In May 2008 Solvay and class-action litigants in California agreed to a settlement of $30 million.[62] Litigants outside California were awarded $16.5 million two years later.[63]

In March 2009, Solvay Pharmaceuticals announced it would discontinue supplying pharmacies with Estratest[64] and by mid-2010, many other producers of generic esterified oestrogen and methyltestosterone products had also discontinued production.[65]

Despite the lawsuits and lack of FDA approval, formulations of esterified oestrogens and methyltestosterone are still available off-label and are still being prescribed to menopausal women. Products available in the US include Covaryx, Essian and EEMT.

Tibolone

Not to be confused with Toblerone, tibolone is not a testosterone product but a synthetic steroid which has oestrogenic effects. Branded as Livial, it is prescribed in 90 countries to treat menopausal symptoms and 45 countries to prevent osteoporosis,[66] including Australia and the UK. Research has found that tibolone can activate the progesterone and androgen receptors and increase circulating free testosterone.[67]

In the US tibolone was rejected by the FDA in 2006 after it was found to double the risk of ischaemic stroke in women over 60 years.[68] This research also found that tibolone may be associated with a slightly increased risk of endometrial cancer.

Esme Nijland (2008) found that tibolone improved sexual wellbeing in postmenopausal women with low libido. They had greater improvements in desire, arousal, satisfaction and receptiveness than did women receiving transdermal oestrogen-progestin therapy.[69]

In a review of clinical trials, Margaret Wierman concluded that tibolone is effective in the treatment of menopausal symptoms, vaginal atrophy and improved sexual function for many women but the benefits need to be balanced against the risks.[70] Susan Davis and Esme Nijland suggest that postmenopausal women with female sexual dysfunction should try tibolone therapy before trying testosterone with or without oestrogen therapy.[71]

DHEA therapy

It has been proposed that because dehydroepiandrosterone (DHEA) and its sulfate, DHEAS, are important precursors for oestrogen and androgen production, treatment with DHEA might help relieve hormone deficiency symptoms in postmenopausal women.

While a number of small studies from 1999 to 2006 indicated benefits from DHEA supplementation,[72] experts now challenge the quality of those studies and the claimed benefits of DHEA.

In 2011 Susan Davis and her colleagues summarised the physiology of DHEA in women and reviewed the findings from randomised placebo controlled trials of the effects of DHEA therapy in postmenopausal women.[73] They found that while these studies indicated a link between low DHEA levels and impaired sexual function and wellbeing in postmenopausal women, the trials did not show that oral DHEA helped relieve these conditions. They concluded that the trial outcomes did not support the use of DHEA in postmenopausal women.

For women with adrenal insufficiency, Margaret Wierman found that the majority of clinical trials of DHEA replacement showed no benefits for sexual function.[74]

The DHEA and Well-ness (DAWN) study led by Donna Kritz-Silverstein in 2008 found that while DHEA supplementation for healthy older men and women restored youthful DHEA levels and enhanced oestrogens and testosterone in women, there were no benefits for sexual function or mood.[75]

The DHEA story is a lesson in not jumping to conclusions, especially when research findings are published in the mass media—as they increasingly often are. It often takes a number of high-quality studies to show the efficacy or otherwise of any therapy.

Data emerging from well-designed trials appear to support the benefits of testosterone supplementation for aspects of female sexual function especially for women who have undergone surgical menopause or have hypopituitarism or adrenal insufficiency. Yet this is within the context of industry promotion, and we still do now know the *long-term* risks of testosterone supplementation. The case is even less clear for premeonpausal women who have been diagnosed with HSDD.

We have to be cautious. As we saw with HRT, the benefits to women were touted well before long-term follow-up was available. There is a risk that testosterone therapy may have a similar storyline—what starts off promising relief may end up delivering sickness in many cases. It's premature to make a general recommendation about testosterone replacement in older women with low testosterone. As with so much about female sexuality, we just don't know.

Sex drugs: the central nervous system

There have been numerous failed attempts at gaining approval for drugs that are claimed to alter our brain chemistry and turn us into sexual Stepford Wives. But some companies have been more persistent than others.

Flibanserin

Flibanserin, mentioned in Chapter 6, is the chemical baby of a German drug maker Boehringer Ingelheim (BI). It acts on the central nervous system by hitting several circuits in the brain that are linked to feelings and pleasure. The FDA views drugs that affect the complicated central nervous system with extra caution. Good thing, that.

In the late 1990s, BI found that flibanserin seemed to relieve stress in rats; however, it failed as an antidepressant in human trials. The company surveyed patients in its clinical trial to assess low libido and found that although there were no improvements in mood, many of the women reported a surge in sexual desire and arousal. This resulted in four major clinical trials, involving 5000 women in 220 locations. In other words, a lot of money and a lot of hype.

The effects of the drug were not immediate. BI spokesman Mark R. Vincent said: 'This is not something that can be taken on a Friday for the weekend . . . There is a gradual increase in sexual desire over a six to eight-week period.'[76]

The FDA panel agreed that those who took the drug did experience a slight increase in sexually satisfying events, but found that there was no proof that it increased their desire. Further, side effects such as dizziness and nausea and concerns about interactions with other drugs, led the FDA to reject flibanserin in June 2010. Although it's easy to dismiss flibanserin as a dud, like many drugs, it may resurrect itself in the future. Refashioned, of course.

Bupropion (Zyban)

Bupropion was approved by the FDA as an antidepressant in 1985, and reintroduced in 1989 after the original dose was found to cause seizures. In 1997, the drug was also approved in the US as a smoking cessation aid. It is currently approved in Australia, the US and many other countries as an antidepressant or smoking cessation aid. But it has started to reveal another unexpected benefit: efficacy in treating HSDD in premenopausal women. Doctors now prescribe it off-label for this purpose. Although bupropion has the lowest incidence of sexual adverse effects when used as an antidepressant, its overall record as a prosexual therapeutic agent is less consistent.

Several studies indicate that bupropion relieves sexual dysfunction in people who do not have depression. For example, in a double-blind study, 63 per cent of men and women on a 12-week course of bupropion rated their condition as much improved or very much improved, versus 3 per cent of those taking a placebo.[77] In two papers by Robert Segraves and his colleagues, one of which was placebo-controlled, bupropion was shown to improve arousal, orgasm and overall satisfaction in women with HSDD.[78] Another study also showed positive effects on orgasmic dysfunction.[79]

Despite side effects—skin reactions, psychiatric disturbances, problems involving the nervous system and gastrointestinal tract—bupropion, or fine-tuned pharmaceutical like it, shows promise as a future brain drug to 'improve' female sexuality.

Bremelanotide

Bremelanotide has the potential to become an international habit. In over 2000 patients who have received its drug, maker Palatin Technologies reports demonstrated reductions of both erectile dysfunction and female sexual dysfunction. Double whammy.

Formerly 'PT-141', bremelanotide is a synthetic drug that activates the melanocortin receptors in the central nervous system, triggering increased sexual desire and genital arousal. It began its bizarre life as melanotan II, a sunless 'tanning' drug nicknamed 'the Barbie drug'. Side effects of mild nausea and a 'stretching and yawning complex' were accompanied by spontaneous penile erections.

Thinking they were onto something, the researchers did another study on men with erectile dysfunction. They alternated doses of melanotan II with a placebo in ten men: nine of them developed erections when given the real drug. In an interview with CNN in 1999, the study head, Hunter Wessells, said the erections happened effortlessly: 'These men were not looking at erotic video tapes. They weren't engaging in sexual activity. They were just sitting around. And on the placebo, none of them got any erectile activity—zero.'[80] The researchers concluded that 'Melanotan II is a potent initiator of erections in men with psychogenic erectile dysfunction and has manageable side effects.'[81] This finding was reinforced by another study of 20 men.[82]

Palatin Technologies developed PT-141, a nasal spray, from melanotan II. It was rejected by the FDA in 2007 after phase II clinical trials showed an unacceptable risk of high blood pressure. In 2008 Palatin backed away from PT-141, but the following year it resumed efforts to get approval for trials of a subcutaneous (under skin) form of the drug. Bremelanotide was born.

In August 2010 Palatin reported positive results for its phase I clinical trial of bremelanotide to treat erectile dysfunction and female sexual dysfunction. The FDA approved further research on the basis that there was no sign the drug caused increased blood pressure. Palatin expected to meet with the FDA to discuss starting a phase II study of the drug both alone and in combination with a PDE-5 inhibitor such as sildenafil (Viagra).

While most of the excitement about bremelanotide has been about spontaneous hard-ons, what might it be able to provide women? A 2004 study by psychologist James Pfaus and his colleagues showed that bremelanotide evoked behaviours in female rats that resembled sexual arousal. Normally in rat sex studies, researchers look for lordosis— when a female rat arches her back in anticipation of the male entering. While subcutaneous injection of bremelanotide did *not* induce lordosis in the female rats, it did increase solicitation behaviours towards male rats.[83] Palatin researchers leapt upon this result.

What is the effect of the drug on human females? A study looked at the effect of bremelanotide on sexual response in 18 premenopausal women with sexual arousal disorder. After a single dose of bremelanotide nasal spray, watching erotic videos did not increase blood flow to their vaginas. However, the women reported increased genital arousal and a statistically significant increase in desire after taking the drug. Also, those who had intercourse within the following 24-hour period were more satisfied with their subjective level of arousal than were those who were given a placebo.[84] So maybe we're not too different from rats after all.

Will a drug like bremelanotide take the hard work out of achieving authentic sexual happiness? Sex writer Leonore Tiefer believes not. 'Sorry, it's never going to happen,' she says. In the meantime, she suggests, there will always be some 'promising' new treatment.[85]

Only four decades ago, the contraceptive pill triggered a sexual revolution, transforming the sex lives of women and men across the world. HRT took this further for women in their post-reproductive years. Men then received the gift of Viagra. Although there is currently no simple pill or patch to safely increase female libido, given the money and effort being expended, it's probably only a matter of time.

We have entered the age of hormone engineering. The pill, HRT, bioidenticals, testosterone therapy, tibolone . . . We improve these drugs by experimenting on willing trial participants—the ageing and the ill, the menopausal, those suffering from hypopituitarism, the adrenally deficient and those labelled as having hypoactive sexual desire disorder (HSDD). When there is enough positive research to prove a drug has benefits that outweigh the risks, government approval is granted. But well before this, a busy trade is already taking place. When drug manufacturers cobble together enough positive research findings to generate excitement, and promote the drug in less stringent countries, an off-label market springs up.

Reflecting a culture that treats symptoms rather than causes, the future will likely see us continuing to take drugs that affect our blood flow, our hormones and our brain chemistry. Many doctors seem to prescribe what their paying patients want. A pill, as they say, for every ill: to boost health and mood, to alleviate pain, to fend off ageing. And, of course, to enhance desire.

Sexual-medicine practitioners and researchers are certainly determined to broaden the range of pharmaceutical treatments available for 'sexually dysfunctional women'. On the last page of Irwin Goldstein and his team's epic 760-page textbook *Women's Sexual Function and Dysfunction: Study, Diagnosis and Treatment*, they share their ultimate goal: 'We look forward to the future when the biologically focused health-care clinician has more pharmaceutical agents available with high levels of robust evidence supporting their safe and effective use in women with sexual health problems.'[86]

Spiritual and religious use of drugs has been occurring since the dawn of our species. Some religions are even based on the use of drugs. Perhaps, one day, sex drugs for women will provide a similar pathway to transcendence.

The difference is, we'll have to pay for it—and it'll be some pharmaceutical company thanking the gods.

10

Bringing sexy back

In most cases, the advice given to women with low libido is to talk to their doctor. But this is the last thing many end up doing. By and large, having a low libido is something a woman resigns herself to. She may feel bad about it from time to time, especially in terms of her partner's frustration. She might have a sense of missing out on an important part of life. But usually, she gets on with things and experiences only occasional jabs of discontent.

Other women take their concern a step further. They do some home research and consult self-help books. They talk to their partners to try to find ways to reconnect, such as watching or reading erotica or planning 'date nights'.

At this point a small minority of women seek treatment. They may try acupuncture, herbal remedies, or sexuality workshops. The success of these types of therapies varies, although some women report significant improvement. And really, besides cash, what is there to lose?

Other women go to their doctor. The doctor has a rather lot to figure out, usually in less than 18 minutes (in the US), or 15 to 20 minutes (in Australia). She will ask about medical history, hormonal status, changes in sexual interest, troubles with arousal, orgasm or vaginal dryness, pain, emotional distress, and use of medications or supplements. Essentially the doctor will try to decide whether the problem relates to libido, arousal, or orgasm difficulties, and whether this is primary (lifelong, having always been this way) or secondary/acquired.

She may perform a pelvic exam, checking for thinning of genital tissues, vaginal dryness or pain-triggering spots, any of which could contribute to a lowered libido. She may recommend thyroid testing. Additionally, and this is where we get into murky ground, the doctor may use 'screening tests' or questionnaires to help her assess the patient's level of desire and determine whether it is 'normal'.

If a screening test reveals a persistent or recurrent lack of sexual thoughts or receptivity to sexual activity which causes personal distress, the patient may be diagnosed with a sexual dysfunction. As discussed in Chapter 9, the doctor may prescribe sex drugs, which affect blood flow, hormone balance or brain chemistry.

Less controversially, at the end of the visit, the doctor may refer the woman to a specialist—a sex therapist or marital counsellor. Relationship issues are a very common underlying cause of loss of desire, and counselling may help.

I once read that sexual problems fit into three basic categories: can't get it up, can't get it in, or can't be bothered. It is possible that talking with a sex therapist or counsellor (with experience in the area of sexuality) will remedy some sexual difficulties. Sex therapy is well recognised for helping women experience orgasms and men get better control of ejaculation. Unfortunately, however, mismatched desire and female low libido persist as the hardest areas to treat. When a woman's interest in sex has never been very strong, it is unlikely that therapy or hormone treatment will dramatically increase her sex drive.

Therapy usually involves education about sexual response, sex techniques and sex homework. Generally treatment involves 4 to 6 months of weekly one-hour sessions. In the US, costs range from $75 to $175 an hour, and in Australia, they are at the higher end of this range. The problem is that when it comes to treating low female desire, sex or marital therapy doesn't have a terribly good success rate.

Countering sexual inertia

Our culture tells us that we deserve more. The TV shows and movies we've watched since we were little girls and boys promise us a life of adventure, and, of course, everlasting—*passionate*—love.

But just as couples come together, so too do they disunite. Our society is one of serial monogamy. Absent the tangy bloom of early courtship and seduction, we are often left with tired couples with unmet needs and mismatched libidos.

Could the shift in desire simply be a result of the ebb and flow of monogamy, the preoccupations of family life and domesticity, the way our bodies, at least women's bodies, were designed? And if that is the case, isn't it perhaps unrealistic to expect that we should have an ever-robust libido when, after all, science reveals that desire tends to dissipate as we age?

Many men and women find themselves in relationships in which libidos are off kilter. That creates a predicament, for discordant desire has a way of undermining even the healthiest and most loving couples. If this is your situation, you may ask, *Who in the relationship is in the best position to fix the sexual stalemate?* Is it you? Is it him?

Why not think about love the way we think about the laws of motion? Here is Newton's first law: *An object's inertia causes it to continue moving at the same speed and in the same direction unless it is acted upon by an unbalanced force.* Inertia, then, means resistance to change. If the forces on us are balanced—that is, in equilibrium—change will not occur.

Inertia is also what happens in long-term relationships, which start off heady and intoxicating, but over time drain themselves of passion. We can counter the sexual stalemate, but the wider is the sexual gap between partners, the greater is the *unbalanced force* that needs to be applied. The more established the pattern, the greater the distance one must bridge. It seems that the longer we stand in the space of lovers turned friends, or lover punishing lover—the longer we stand apart and the greater the work required to restore eros.

Work? Yes.

Whoever said that love and desire would be as easy and plentiful as grass?

Oh that's right, Hollywood did, with her white-veil fantasies and fluorescent smile. But Hollywood forgot to tell you that finding love isn't the hardest battle. Maintaining it is.

Maintaining *jouissance*, spark and eros is difficult. After all, we are working against inertia, against nature. Marrying for love is a twentieth-century Western phenomenon. *And we are scriptless*, left on open terrain without signposts to direct us to adult desire.

If you are in a relationship where the sexual current has slowed, an important question to ask is, *Who has the most to lose if the situation is not improved?* If desire remains dormant, with one partner unsatisfied, what might the consequences be? Marital incompatibility? Threat of adultery? Relationship discontinuation? Or simply one or both of you feeling undesired, unseen?

When men cheat, it is often so that they can be *seen* differently—as important, powerful, sexy, exciting, larger than they are in the four walls of their home relationship. Women, too, may look to a new lover to be heard, witnessed, appreciated. It is this freshness that gives an affair voltage. At its heart, an affair is highly narcissistic—more about *you* than the other person.

The nature of adult sexuality is still uncertain. It is not known whether we are quasi-monogamous or quasi-polygamous. But throughout time and across cultures, men have found the answer to marital boredom in the arms of an intoxicating—and usually younger—other. Extramarital sex, affairs, prostitutes, mistresses, or even second or third wives, have been almost the norm for the human male.

Even now in many cultures men are not expected to remain faithful to one woman. In fact, the more powerful a man is—or handsome, or charismatic, or rich—the less likely it is thought to be that he'll remain constant. In France, for example, it's considered natural for a powerful man to have an insatiable libido, and he would not necessarily be blamed for exercising it. A wife may look the other way, or start a dalliance of her own, *n'est-ce pas*? Indeed, many European, Asian and African countries have incorporated infidelity into their sociological structure.

And yet, as a general rule, in the West, we do not accept that a man should have other lovers. Our man is ours alone. Departure of his affections is the greatest affront, the greatest betrayal, with divorce a common response. But do we acknowledge our own betrayal—that we may well have denied him sensual intimacies, stopped being his lover long before he started looking elsewhere? Chronically not in the mood ourselves, we tell him he cannot have us, nor can he have anyone else. We demand he be sexually faithful in this our mostly sexless marriage: be sexually mine, but without my physicality, without body love.

That's not to say that in the enterprise of sex and love women aren't also disadvantaged. Most of this book has been about the obstacles to female eros. We are not pretty enough or rested enough, we have a eco chic house to keep up, children to raise, a career to fortify, and wrinkles to control.

When did our dreams become so grand? Can we vanquish our larger-than-life expectations and learn how to be as we are? Learn how to become in tune with whatever stage we're currently in, and accept the sexual implications—whether we are young and experimental, partnered with small children, or menopausal?

Adultery is the primary disrupter of families and the most universally accepted reason for divorce.[1] Given that affairs operate in secrecy, statistics concerning infidelity are highly unreliable. Nevertheless, researchers believe that about half of couples are unfaithful. Men historically have been more adulterous, but women are starting to catch up.[2]

Returning to our earlier question, *Who in the relationship is in the best position to fix the sexual stalemate?* You are. You decided to commit to this person. It is likely that lust once resided between you. It is possible to get it back, to reclaim eros and replenish your sensual relationship.

If our sexual relationship falters, it's up to one person to make the first move, to inject energy, to surprise the other using unbalanced force, to upturn the everyday rituals of domesticity and shift the gridlock of sexlessness. An easy way to begin this is simply to kiss.

Kiss your partner every day. This can keep your sensual bond alive, preventing you from becoming more flatmates than lovers. One kiss doesn't take time. But the pay-off is significant. Kissing sexually, with an open mouth, says, *You are more than a companion to me, more than a friend, we are sensual, in this together.*

From these tiny X-rated kisses, other surprises may develop.

The thing with sex is that once it is resumed, once estranged bed partners have reconnected, a sensual gravity of sorts often draws you back down together. Your bodies like the comfort, the closeness. They want more. Wrangling sex into the domestic front after a long absence can be difficult. But the sensual pulse doesn't take that long to revive, and the effort reaps rewards.

And yet, the initial steps—the planning, the seducing, the facing rejection, the moving beyond waiting for spontaneous desire—hold many back from attempting sensual intimacy. And while desires are held back, swallowed whole, new desires can form . . . for others, for a different life, for a place where one is simultaneously understood, appreciated and adored. You may not realise it, being too busy paying bills and putting sunscreen on toddlers' noses, but your relationship is under threat.

Sexual mindfulness and Tantric libidos

Orgasms originate between the ears, not the legs. Paraplegic or quadriplegic people who have no sensation below the waist can still experience orgasm when their chest or neck is stimulated. Other researchers have found that the brainwaves of women having intense vaginal orgasms mirror those of people deep in meditation.[3]

Tantric philosophy can help revitalise libido. Our knowledge of Tantra is derived from ancient Taoist, Hindu and Buddhist texts and teachings passed down from gurus to students. Today's practitioners have simplified the Tantric canon and created a Westernised version of Tantric yoga, sometimes dubbed 'neo-Tantra' or 'California Tantra'.

As with all yogas, the basic goal of Tantra is to experience union with the divine. In the case of Tantra, this happens when lovers have simultaneous ecstatic sexual experiences. All Tantric exercises are geared towards this ultimate outcome, although on the surface many of them appear to veer in the opposite direction. For instance, in some exercises partners practise touching each other with love while consciously eschewing the intention of arousing sexual desire. Tantra helps counter the mind–body disconnect and teaches us to honour our sexuality.

If taking a tantric workshop or following a tantric book seems too esoteric as a path to reclaiming authentic female pleasure, sex therapists offer some seemingly simple advice: relax. Lower your sexual expectations. Spend less time observing what is happening during sex. And try to be fully engaged in the moment.

Therapist Lori Brotto believes sexual mindfulness may be one of the greatest keys to unlocking libido. It refers to a state of sexual stillness—of being present in the sexual moment. In Brotto's workshops with women, one of their first tasks is . . . balancing an egg on a tabletop. Yep. Brotto has her participants do this because it entails mindfulness—total, singular concentration. Slowly building on this and other techniques, she helps women learn how to be 'present', and then apply this focus in sexual encounters.

Sensuality, particularly for women, is often about our mindset. If there isn't enough space in our mind to entertain erotic sensibilities, then forget about entertaining an actual penis. Learning what exactly makes us feel sensual is the key to everything.

One of the secrets to resuming sex, to bringing it back to forefront, is to turn off The List. We need to learn the most effective way to shut down its voice.

Will getting out of the house in a dress that you love help you remember a feeling of dalliance? Book a babysitter and go out somewhere fanciful: an ice rink, a river bed.

Are you a hot-bath-and-massage kind of woman? Have him run the water for you, wash your hair, dry you the way he dries your children, careful to pat each crevice. And then touch you slowly. Touch you without wanting anything back.

If we can set it up so we feel both attractive and relaxed and are in an environment free of any reminder of chores, half the battle is won. The List has been temporarily filed. Take advantage of its absence. Move slowly. Trick yourself into unwinding, unfolding.

Our desire should not rest on the laurels of another. To build libido, experience desire, and explore our sensuality, we need to create time for self-pleasure in our lives. This could mean setting aside a time when you apply creams to your body in a sensual ritual. A time when you feel your hips, thighs and breasts and reflect upon things that make you feel sexual and beautiful and connected to your body. Slip some erotic poems into your reading. Give sensuality a proper place in your home and learn what turns you on.

Open-eyed libido

We are told that our eyes are the windows to our soul and that through looking at one another we can connect and reveal our most authentic self. But why is it that when we make love our eyes are almost invariably shut; why is it that when we are supposedly the most intimate, maintaining eye-to-eye contact is frankly uncomfortable?

The way we make love is not a biological act; in many ways, it is cultural, with associated scripts. With my Spanish boyfriend Antonio, I was shocked the first time we had sex. Not only did he look directly into my eyes the *entire* time, he also uttered declarations throughout, such as *mi poco se zambulló* (my little dove), and *mi reina* (my queen). Not typical Commonwealth bedroom behaviour, as I'm sure you'll agree.

When it comes to sex, we look at each other in different ways, but rarely eye-to-eye. We look at each other with an objectifying gaze, at which men are particularly practised, depersonalising and treating the other as a sex object. This isn't necessarily always a bad thing; such a gaze can heat up an encounter and give it pulse. There is also the self-defeating gaze, where we clock an inventory of our sexual weaknesses—that we are not big enough, small enough, good enough. I know numerous women who insist on making love with the lights off. They don't want their partners to see them naked. They don't want to see themselves naked. And then there are those of us who glance at our partner's body or, daringly, his face during sex. To spy our partner caught in rapture feels exciting, like trespassing upon his privacy, and then, when he catches us looking, and our eyes meet, there is a charge, a rush. But one person usually looks away. The feeling of exposure is too much.

According to *Passionate Marriage* author David Schnarch, this is precisely the time when we should try to maintain eye contact. Instead of tuning into one another during sex, Schnarch believes we tune out and focus on the sensations of our body. In his workshops he jokes that one of the reasons many of us don't like to masturbate is because we find it lonely; most of us prefer sex with someone else, so we can ignore them.

Schnarch writes: 'Our anatomical ability to sustain eye contact during face-to-face intercourse facilitates our uniquely human capacity for intimacy during sex. And yet couples ignore how vision taps into out innate emotional connection with other humans.'[4]

Often in foreplay we get stuck within a particular pattern, driven by the same emotional intent. Using the eyes-open method can change the ambience of sex.

Open-eyed kissing, open-eyed foreplay, open-eyed sex and for those over-achievers, open-eyed orgasm provide a pathway to erotic sex. Eastern tradition is well aware of this. In Eastern approaches to sexuality, it's not unusual for partners to look directly into each other's eyes during sexual encounters.

New York psychologist Arthur Arun conducted an experiment with a group of men and women. Putting opposite-sex pairs—previously perfect strangers—in rooms together, he instructed each pair to perform a series of tasks and then had each couple stare into each other's eyes for a number of minutes without talking. Afterwards, many of his couples reported feeling deeply attracted to their study pair, and one of his ad-hoc 'couples' eventually got married.

Being 'I-open', Schnarch believes, can help us see what is lying beneath the surface of our relationship, make familiar sex foreign, stay in the present, increase differentiation and 'tolerance for intimacy and passion' and, ultimately, use sexuality in order to see the self. And if you think about it, what's the point of being face-to-face if we keep our eyes shut? To see and be seen. Oh, the thrill.

Prioritising passion

Despite their unprecedentedly busy lives, women have a lot of time for passion. It's just that after a relationship has been established, the passion they find themselves focusing on can be less about eroticism and more about passionate mothering, having a passionate career, passionate home and food presentation, or a passion-inducing appearance.

If you find your sexual desire is lacking and you wish to reclaim it, energy must be removed from other areas of your life. Something has to give. A sober look at how you divide your time may help give a sense of where to place adult sensuality and what shortcuts to take. For instance: *Domestic*—Does your pumpkin soup need to be homemade? A can of soup will save an extra hour of your day that can be devoted to creating a sensual space for yourself. *Mothering*—Are you expending more energy on raising your children than on nurturing your marriage? If so, what small acts can you perform to reverse this imbalance? For example, although some mothers boycott children's television programs, using such media can grant you some quality time with your partner on weekend mornings. *Appearance*— Instead of spending our time attempting to look desirable, let's *be* desirable. Let's skip the pretence of looking sexy and instead explore how to be sexy, in whatever way suits us best.

Making sensual living a part of daily or weekly life gives it room to expand and find itself. It, like many things, involves a decision. To create a more sensual life, we need to allow time and space for sexuality to feel its way into shape. Creating an environment where libido can emerge, where you can affirm the importance of your partner and reconnect to yourself as a sexual woman, enables your relationship to maintain eroticism. This involves creating a bedroom that complements relaxation, freshness and desire and a weekly schedule that has spaces in it.

Setting aside time for intimacy may come across as contrived and boring, but if intimacy is not consciously made room for, desire might not make house calls. It's time we got over our discomfort with planned intimacy and stopped being so precious. Anticipation is one of the greatest igniters of desire, and by engineering a little intimacy we can enjoy the *lead-up* to sex and its inherent erotic tension. Scheduling time for just the two of you gives eros priority. And eros likes that.

A popular method of rekindling romance and strengthening the marital bond is to schedule weekly or monthly date nights. Hereupon the haggard couple take time to dine out and, removed from the domestic, give sexual identity a chance to rediscover itself.

Manufacturing danger and distance

Another way to uproot romantic ennui is to stimulate chemical production. If it's rollercoaster love you're after, try rollercoaster activities. It has been found that when we encounter danger, our biochemical arousal response can also be activated. This is why sex therapists often encourage rock climbing. Seriously.

Arthur Aron's research revealed that novelty incites dopamine production, heightening feelings of attraction. Apparently even jogging on the spot and then meeting a potential partner increases the likelihood of being attracted to them—yet another reason to feel bad about not exercising. A different experiment showed that if people experience fear on a date, they often misinterpret it as love. Attraction is heightened under anxiety-provoking circumstances, and these heightened feelings can be misdirected to the most suitable target.[5] Doing new or dangerous things with your partner boosts adrenaline. Activities that may provide a jolt to relationships turned lacklustre can range from a wee bit new to . . . spanking new, literally.

Another way to help keep a relationship robust is to manufacture a degree of separation. Much of Esther Perel's book *Mating in Captivity,* for example, explores how intimacy can in fact repel eros.[6] For Perel, true emotional, psychological and physical differentiation is at the heart of keeping long-term relationships sexually dynamic. This is reminiscent of Lacan's *jouissance*, discussed in Chapter 5. We are psychologically wired to chase that which we cannot attain and we get off on the pleasure and pain of separation. It fuels our desire. Close relationships have a tendency to smother this dynamic. To tap into our *jouissance* and that of our partners, a little unbalanced force may be in order.

We can create physical and emotional separation by going on holidays by ourself or with friends, taking night classes, or pouring ourselves into projects outside the domain of the home. Emotionally we can look to others to confide in sometimes and have deep relationships with, to keep our primary relationship fresh, alluring and full of new currents.

Another more intensive strategy is to explore your core erotic motif, as detailed in the fascinating book *The Erotic Mind* by psychotherapist Jack Morin. Morin believes that the emotional difficulties faced in childhood often serve as building blocks for adult desire; that old wounds and conflicts can transform into excitation. By examining our peak sexual experiences, we can uncover our core erotic themes and apply them to our current sexual relationship to uproot sexual listlessness.[7] This book allows us to play sexual detective and learn about our own personalised desire.

Discovering female *jouissance*

As women we have the ability to tap into a form of *jouissance* 'outside sex'. Our sexuality is not limited to that defined by society's objectifying gaze. According to Alan and Donna Brauer, the average orgasm is 10 seconds long and the average frequency of intercourse once or twice a week. This translates to 20 seconds a week, one and a half minutes a month, and about 18 minutes a year. The authors ask us to consider how many thousands of hours we think, worry and daydream about sex when, in a 50-year span, we experience a total of 15 hours of orgasmic ecstasy.[8] But brevity does not to equate to significance.

Good wine, good food, good weather and good sex have a few things in common. They all have an enormous impact on our wellbeing and are major players in the good life.

Apparently, a glass of shiraz can be the equivalent to K-Y Jelly. A 2010 Italian study (and if you were to be in a study, surely this would be the pick) revealed that drinking one or two glasses of red wine each day increases female sexual desire. Among 789 women aged 18 to 50, red wine was found to reduce inhibitions while influencing sexual play.[9] So next time you slip into something more comfortable, sip on something, too.

A romantic meal has long been considered a preliminary to great sex. Indeed, they say the way to a man's heart is through his stomach. Professor Ronald Noë has found this to be so, at least for non-human primates. Noë discovered that monkeys exchange grooming for food and sex. After he trained one female vervet monkey to open a plastic box filled with food, she was rewarded by being groomed more often and for longer by the other monkeys.[10] Reflect on this when next you pack your partner's lunch in a Tupperware container.

Be it food, wine or slinky jazz clubs, it is up to us to discover what turns us on, how we like to make love and be made love to, and when and how we feel sexy. Personalising our own aphrodisiacs and using them to get us in the mood is a liberating way to reclaim our libido. Being able to find our own *jouissance*—to define female pleasure outside of the parameters of patriarchy—will help us creatively explore and construct an authentic sexuality, rather than one that mirrors the false ideals pushed by media and marketing profiteers.

To bring pleasure into our life—both sexually and in terms of spirit and vitality—let us experiment with *jouissance* to find our own true libido.

Conclusion

It began in mystery, and it will end in mystery, but what a savage and beautiful country lies in between.

Diane Ackerman[1]

We are oestrous beings. Our bodies, moods and desires fluctuate with tidal hormones. First in puberty, then in waves of menstrual cycles, for some of us during pregnancy, birthing and breastfeeding, and then in menopause.

Many of us are also sexual victims, having experienced abuse at the hand of someone we know. Alongside our own personal history, we are also situated in a world history of female sexual oppression.

Women, too, are targets of corporate marketers, their thousands of messages whispered to us as though from inside the space of dreaming, *you are not enough*, you do not look desirable enough, you do not desire enough.

Market-driven ideals about beauty affect our libido and often dictate our sense of sexual worth. But the beauty being endorsed does not value motherhood, age, or imperfection. And so we are all left out. Instead of focusing on eros, all we can see is the sexual desirability we feel we do not have, *our lack*, and this is where we channel much of our time, money, and thoughts.

Western women are also by and large believers in the myth of passionate monogamy—that most relationships will be able to accommodate both desire and family, eros and familiarity. Having opened ourselves to love so many times, and having had many of our romantic entanglements end in disappointment, we are heart-sore. Having experienced break-ups, divorce, adultery, or the sadness of living in a relationship that doesn't match the glossy world of Hollywood scripts, we are often left disillusioned.

Given the freedom and transient pleasures of extended youth we imagine a future for ourselves devoid of the mundane. But this is not what we find in long-term monogamy. The two worlds, what we expect our lives to be like and what we actually find it to be like, are dangerously incongruent. They clash. Often this leaves both people in a relationship isolated, sexless, blaming each other.

Indeed, in our era, not to have frequent electrifying sex, is equivalent to not having money or status. Sex has become a value of happiness and success whereby the (mostly) celibate couple is the failed couple. But the fact is, in established relationships women often experience low levels of spontaneous desire. Sex usually declines in priority and frequency.

Let us deconstruct the fairy tale and throw it away for good. As we once got over the idea that Prince Charming would come to rescue us, we now need to deal with the second stage of the myth: family life. Realistically, the loss of freedom, spontaneity, and sex-focus must be acknowledged and from this platform, decisions made about the role of adult desire. What part will eros play in our life? How much effort are we going to put into reclaiming it? Is this a mutual goal? It is up to us to write the script.

Women, too, seem set up to fail, cast to play worker, mother, domestic, wife, friend, and of course, vixen. This has lead to role overload and exhaustion, to guilt and lethargy.

Increasingly we turn to drugs. These drugs alter our melancholy and depression, our menopause, our ageing, and our sexuality. Pharmaceutical companies and the scientists on their bankroll recast sexual disinterest as something altogether more sinister: sexual dysfunction. But as our discussion of sex models past to present revealed, efforts thus far have not identified a successful model of female libido. Women's sex drive remains an unsolved mystery, making 'normal' or 'dysfunctional' definitions impossible.

Medical intervention in the female body is not new. It is becoming commonplace in the areas of reproduction, childbirth, menopause, sexual function and libido, the brain (antidepressants), and in cosmetic surgical procedures. While there is no doubt that the people working in these fields genuinely want to help people who have lost something or lack something, as a whole they tap into a collective psyche that has led us to believe we can always *take control* and buy our way out of trouble. The drugs being trialled and marketed to buttress sex will no doubt eventually offer a panacea for our sexual problems. It is only a matter of time before a pink Viagra arrives on the pharmacy shelves.

And for those of us who feel we are losing the battle, that the obstacles to sexual fulfilment are too overwhelming, this will be a welcome development.

From the Sex Drive thus far, we have learned about libido and the factors that can hinder our desire. We have explored some of the cultural and biological differences between male and female sexuality. Motherhood has been examined as a sensual rival to the romantic pair. The children in our lives have been revamped from being 'seen but not heard' to mini-gods on pedestals, with yummy mummies, who look like sex, but have none.

Menopause and ageing are challenges to our sense of our sexual selves. However, *sexual attitudes* arguably affect our sexual behavior more than the ageing process. Women who give greater priority to sex in their everyday lives are less likely to experience low desire, low orgasmic function and low arousal. Indeed, it seems nothing trumps relationship factors when it comes (or doesn't cum) to low desire. Women's sexual response is greatly influenced by how they feel about their partner, and studies indicate that this may be more important than hormones to sexual response.

And so, if a woman ends up with a healthy vibrant libido no matter what her stage of life, it is almost *despite* her journey as a woman in the world, which works in so many ways to dismantle it. For the few of us that get through these hurdles and still have a libido intact, recognise this accomplishment. As we progress through life's stages having a robust, high libido is the exception not the rule. That's not to say we cannot have a renaissance—after kids, after refinding or recreating ourselves, or meeting that amazing person who makes us feel both completely comfortable and completely alert.

For the rest of us, rather than pathologising 'low libido', it may serve us to say, screw it. Let's embrace our fluctuating, precious and resilient libido, wherever, whenever, in whatever form it manifests. By accepting libido as it presents itself, we change our relationship with it. No longer wishing it to be other than it is, we allow it to come into its own natural form. Armed with knowledge about the elusive nature of female desire and its individual contradictions, we have the power to determine what libido means to us.

Yet we are social creatures who look to our neighbours to determine what is both adequate and desirable. Status anxiety—keeping up with the Joneses (or the Kardashians)—is a human vulnerability and one that companies and their marketing firms are skilled at exploiting. 'Normal' is a powerful term, 'dysfunctional' even more so. There is an assumption that everyone should have the same level of interest in sex, and that level should be high but, as this book shows, gender and culture shape our ideas about what is appropriate sexual behavior. There is a wide spectrum of ways to be sexually healthy, and it is our own satisfaction and our partner's that should concern us.

If we are so inclined, in pursuit of our full sex drive we can engage in sex therapy, drug treatment, Tantra or other mindfulness practices, exploring themes of unbalanced force, creating distance, manufacturing danger, or reprioritising and scheduling sex. But whatever road we choose, let us work towards defining our own *jouissance*, a personalised sensuality in which we are actively sexy rather than seeking sex. After all, sexual prime is a function of 'sexiness'—and *that* can peak at any age.

Endnotes

Introduction

1   EO Laumann et al (1999) 'Sexual dysfunction in the United States: prevalence and predictors', *JAMA*, vol. 281, pp 537–44.
2   R Basson (2005) 'Women's sexual dysfunction: revised and expanded definitions', *Canadian Medical Association Journal*, 10 May, vol. 172, issue 10.
3   D Klusmann (2006) 'Sperm competition and female procurement of male resources as explanations for a sex-specific time course in the sexual motivation of couples', *Journal of Human Nature*, vol. 17, no. 3, pp. 283–300.
4   'Australian women urged to remember you' (2006) *femail.com.au* <www.femail.com.au/remember-you.htm> [accessed January 2011].
5   The names and identifying characteristics of the people who shared their stories with me have been changed.

Chapter 1

1   N Wolf (1991) *The Beauty Myth: How images of beauty are used against women*, Vintage, London.
2   DM Buss (1989) 'Sex differences in human mate preferences: evolutionary hypotheses tested in 37 cultures', *Behavioral and Brain Sciences*, vol. 12, pp. 1–49.

3 R Parker (2010) *Women, Doctors, and Cosmetic Surgery: Negotiating the 'normal' body*, Palgrave Macmillan, UK.

4 T Olds and K Norton (1999) 'How to become a supermodel', paper presented to 'The Body Culture Conference: Challenging current approaches to physical activity, healthy eating, sexual health and body image', Melbourne.

5 S Orbach (1999), 'Whose body? The politics of the body and the body politic', paper presented to 'The Body Culture Conference'.

6 *Encyclopedia of Products & Industries—Manufacturing* (2001) 'Cosmeceuticals', Gale Cengage, first edn.

7 B Delaney (2005) 'The shape of things to come', *Sydney Morning Herald*, <www.smh.com.au/news/Fashion/The-shape-of-things-to-come/2005/01/07/1104832293293.html> [accessed March 2011].

8 R Smithers (2007) 'Beauty industry failing minority ethnic women', *The Guardian*, 15 November, <www.guardian.co.uk/uk/2007/nov/15/race.retail> [accessed 4 April 2008].

9 S Daniells (2006) 'UK women spend big to look better', *Cosmetics design-Europe.com*, <www.cosmeticsdesign-europe.com/Business-Financial/UK-women-spend-big-to-look-better> [accessed 16 October 2011].

10 'Dalai Lama says cosmetics make people look like "creatures from outer space"' (2008) *One India News*, 14 June <http://news.oneindia.in/2008/06/14/dalai-lama-cosmetics-make-creatures-outer-space-1213443180.html> [accessed 16 October 2011].

11 'Archbishop Vikenty of Yekaterinburg asks women to enhance their beauty with prayer rather than with makeup' (2008) *Interfax*, pub 4 February, quoted on *Orthodox England* <www.orthodoxengland.org.uk/makeup.htm> [accessed 4 April 2008].

12 C Comiskey (2004) 'Cosmetic surgery in Paris in 1926: the case of the amputated leg', *Journal of Women's History*, vol. 16, pp. 30–54.

13 'The "Body Beautiful" costs big bucks' (2010) *IBISWorld*, 16 December, <www.ibisworld.com.au/about/media/pressrelease/release.aspx?id=245> [accessed 16 October 2011].

14 R Parker (2010) *Women, Doctors, and Cosmetic surgery: Negotiating the 'normal' body*, Palgrave Macmillan, UK.

15 'ASPS Statistics for Cosmetic Plastic Surgery in the United States' (2009) *Consumer guide to plastic surgery*, <www.yourplasticsurgeryguide.com/trends/asps-2009.htm> [accessed November 2011].

16 '2009 report of the 2008 statistics: national clearinghouse of plastic surgery statistics' (2009) American Society of Plastic Surgeons, <www.plasticsurgery.org/Media/stats/2008-US-cosmetic-reconstructive-plastic-surgery-minimally-invasive-statistics.pdf> [accessed January 2010].

17 Delaney, 'The shape of things to come', <www.smh.com.au/news/Fashion/The-shape-of-things-to-come/2005/01/07/1104832293293.html>.

18 ibid.

19 Parker, *Women, Doctors and Cosmetic Surgery*, pp. 5, 8, 176.

20 A Lingis (1996) 'The body postured and dissolute', in VM Foti (ed.), *Merleau-Ponty: Difference, materiality, painting*, Humanities Press, p. 65.

21 A Schembri (2010) 'Eating Disorders and Obsessive-Compulsive Disorder: An Examination of Overlapping Symptoms, Obsessive Beliefs, and Associated Cognitive Dimensions', PhD thesis, Division of Psychology, School of Health Sciences, College of Science, Engineering, and Health, RMIT University.

22 ibid.

23 R Eckersley (2005) *Well & Good: Morality, meaning and happiness*, second edn, Text, Melbourne, p. 140.

24 G McArthur (2007) 'Not worth weight, girls', *Herald Sun*, 20 July, p. 11.

25 American Psychological Association (2011) 'Sexualization of girls' <www.apa.org/pi/women/programs/girls/report.aspx> [accessed November 2011].

26 S Doonan (2008) *Eccentric Glamour: Creating an insanely more fabulous you*, Simon & Schuster Paperbacks, New York.

27 BL Hankin and L Abramson (2001) 'Development of gender differences in depression: an elaborated cognitive vulnerability-transactional stress theory', *Psychological Bulletin*, vol. 127, pp. 1–40.

28 M McCabe and L Ricciardelli (1999) 'Socio-cultural influences on body image and body change strategies among adolescent boys', paper presented to 'The Body Culture Conference: Challenging current approaches to physical activity, healthy eating, sexual health and body image', Melbourne.

29 S Faludi (1991) *Backlash: The undeclared war against American women*, 15th edn, Three Rivers Press, New York, p. 203.

30 J Richters et al (2003) 'Sex in Australia: sexual difficulties in a representative sample of adults', *Australian and New Zealand Journal of Public Health*, vol. 27, no. 2, pp. 164–70.

31 A Burns (2008) 'Flab, not fab, in bed', *mX*, *Herald Sun*, 28 March, p. 5.

32 BL Fredrickson and TA Roberts (1997) 'Objectification theory: toward understanding women's lived experiences and mental health risks', *Psychology of Women Quarterly*, vol. 21, pp. 173–206.

33 MD Siever (1994) 'Sexual orientation and gender as factors in socioculturally acquired vulnerability to body dissatisfaction and eating disorders', *Journal of Consulting and Clinical Psychology*, vol. 62, no. 2, pp. 252–60.

34 WH Masters and VE Johnson (1970) *Human Sexual Inadequacy*, Little, Brown, Boston.

35 DH Barlow (1986) 'Causes of sexual dysfunction: the role of anxiety and cognitive interference', *Journal of Consulting and Clinical Psychology*, vol. 54, no. 2, pp. 140–8.

36 JW Pennebaker and T Roberts (1992) 'Toward a his and hers theory of emotion: gender differences in visceral perception', *Journal of Social and Clinical Psychology*, vol. 11, no. 3, pp. 199–212; T Roberts and JW Pennebaker (1995) 'Gender differences in perceiving internal state: toward a his-and-hers model of perceptual cue use', *Advances in Experimental Social Psychology*, vol. 27, pp. 143–75.

37 E Laan et al (1995) 'Determinants of subjective experience of sexual arousal in women: feedback from genital arousal and erotic stimulus content', *Psychophysiology*, vol. 32, no. 5, pp. 444–51.

38 HG Pope et al (2001) 'The growing commercial value of the male body: a longitudinal survey of advertising in women's magazines', *Psychotherapy and Psychosomatics*, vol. 70, pp. 189–92.

39 Wolf, *The Beauty Myth*, p. 277.

40 J Ropelato 'Internet pornography statistics', *TopTenReviews* <http://internet-filter-review.toptenreviews.com/internet-pornography-statistics.html#time> [accessed 29 April 2008].

41   AM Elliott and CC Lemert (2005) *The New Individualism: The emotional costs of globalization*, Rowman & Littlefield, London.

Chapter 2

1   'Sex does the body good: regular romps can provide a host of physiological benefits' (2006) *Forbes.com*, 19 December, <www.msnbc.msn.com/id/16282622/ns/health-forbes_com/t/sex-does-body-good/#.TpobF81fy2w> [accessed November 2011].

2   S Ebrahim et al (2002) 'Sexual intercourse and risk of ischaemic stroke and coronary heart disease: the Caerphilly study', *J Epidemiol Community Health*, vol. 56, pp. 99–102.

3   G Giles et al (2003) 'Sexual factors and prostate cancer', *BJU International*, vol. 92, issue 3, pp. 211–16.

4   M Leitzmann et al (2004) 'Ejaculation frequency and subsequent risk of prostate cancer', *JAMA*, vol. 291, no. 13, pp. 1578–86.

5   Gouin et al (2010) 'Marital behavior, oxytocin, vasopressin, and wound healing', *Psychoneuroendocrinology*, August, vol. 35, issue 7, pp. 1082–90, <www.ncbi.nlm.nih.gov/pubmed/20144509> [accessed May 2011].

6   CJ Charnetski and FX Brennan (2004) 'Sexual frequency and salivary immunoglobulin A (IgA)', *Psychological Reports*, vol. 94, no. 3, pp. 839–44.

7   'Church challenge: have sex every day' (2008) *Sydney Morning Herald*, <www.smh.com.au/articles/2008/02/20/1203190867062.html> [accessed June 2011].

8   YR Avellanet et al (2008) 'Relationship between loss of libido and signs and symptoms of depression in a sample of Puerto Rican middle-aged women', *Puerto Rico Health Sciences Journal*, vol. 27, no. 1, pp. 85–91; EO Laumann et al (1999) 'Sexual Dysfunction in the United States: Prevalence and predictors', *JAMA*, vol. 281, no. 6, pp. 537–44.

9   RM Abu Ali et al (2008) 'Sexual dysfunction in Jordanian diabetic women', *Diabetics Care*, vol. 31, no. 8, pp. 1580–1; J Miocić, N Car and Z Metelko (2008) 'Sexual dysfunction in women with diabetes mellitus', *Diabetologia Croatica*, vol. 37, no. 2, pp. 35–42.

10 S Davis (2006) 'Available therapies and outcome results in premenopausal women' in *Women's Sexual Function and Dysfunction: Study, diagnosis and treatment*, Taylor & Francis, London and New York, p. 545.

11 'Australian women urged to remember you' (2006) *femail.com.au*, <www.femail.com.au/remember-you.htm> [accessed January 2011].

12 'Top ten things better than sex' (2010) *TopTenz.net* <www.toptenz.net/top-10-things-better-than-sex.php> [accessed October 2011].

13 D Klusmann (2006) 'Sperm competition and female procurement of male resources as explanations for a sex-specific time course in the sexual motivation of couples', *Journal of Human Nature*, vol. 17, no. 3, pp. 283–300.

14 J Borneman and LK Hart (2004) 'An elastic institution: the natural evolution of marriage', *The Washington Post*, 14 April, p. A25.

15 Z Bauman (2000) *Liquid Modernity*, Polity Press, Cambridge, UK.

16 L Vandervoot and S Duck (2004) 'Sex, lies, and ... transformation', in J Duncombe (ed.), *The State of Affairs: Explorations in infidelity and commitment*, Lawrence Eribaum Associates, Nahwah, NJ, pp. 1–14.

17 R King (2006) 'Doctor, where did my libido go?', *O&G*, vol. 8, no. 3, pp. 9–10.

18 ibid.

19 ibid.

20 JK McNulty and TD Fisher (2008) 'Gender differences in response to sexual expectancies and changes in sexual frequency: a short-term longitudinal study of sexual satisfaction in newly married couples', *Archives of Sexual Behavior*, vol. 37, pp. 229–40.

21 BP Acevedo and A Aron (2009) 'Does a long-term relationship kill romantic love?', *Review of General Psychology*, vol. 13, no. 1, pp. 59–65.

22 ES Byers (2005) 'Relationship satisfaction and sexual satisfaction: a longitudinal study of individuals in long-term relationships', *The Journal of Sex Research*, vol. 42, no. 2, pp. 113–18.

23 D Holmberg and KL Blair (2009) 'Sexual desire, communication, satisfaction, and preferences of men and women in same-sex

versus mixed-sex relationships', *Journal of Sex Research*, vol. 46, no. 1, pp. 57–66.

24 M Nichols (2006) 'Sexual function in women with women: lesbians and lesbian relationships', in I Goldstein et al (eds) *Women's Sexual Function and Dysfunction: Study, diagnosis, and treatment*, Taylor and Francis, London and New York, p. 12.

25 RT Michael et al (1995) *Sex in America: A definitive survey*, Little, Brown, Boston.

26 V Call and P Schwartz (1995) 'The incidence and frequency of marital sex in a national sample', *Journal of Marriage and Family*, vol. 57, no. 3, pp. 639–52.

27 JR Heiman, SJ Long, SN Smith, WA Fisher, MS Sand and RC Rosen (2011) 'Sexual satisfaction and relationship happiness in midlife and older couples in five countries', *Archives of Sexual Behavior*, vol. 40, pp. 741–53.

28 'Sexual wellbeing global survey' (2008) Durex <www.durex.com/en-US/SexualWellbeingSurvey/pages/default.aspx> [accessed 27 January 2011].

29 M Weiner-Davis (2003) *The Sex-starved Couple: A couple's guide to boosting their marriage libido*, Simon & Schuster, New York.

30 DA Donnelly and EO Burgess (2008) 'The decision to remain in an involuntarily celibate relationship', *Journal of Marriage and Family*, vol. 70, no. 3, pp. 519–35.

Chapter 3

1 DP Schmitt et al (2002) 'Is there an early-30s peak in female sexual desire? Cross-sectional evidence from the United States and Canada', *The Canadian Journal of Human Sexuality*, vol. 11, no. 1, p. 14.

2 A Barr, A Bryan and D Kenrick (2002) 'Sexual peak: socially shared cognitions about desire, frequency and satisfaction in men and women', *Personal Relationships*, vol. 9, no. 3, pp. 287–99.

3 RR Baker and MA Bellis (1995) *Human Sperm Competition: Copulation, masturbation and infidelity*, Chapman & Hall, London.

4 M Patel, C Brown and G Bachmann (2006) 'Sexual function in the menopause and perimenopause', in I Goldstein et al (eds)

Women's Sexual Function and Dysfunction: Study, diagnosis and treatment Taylor & Francis, London and New York, p. 253.

5 S Davis (2006) 'Available therapies and outcome results in premenopausal women', *Women's Sexual Function and Dysfunction: Study, diagnosis and treatment*, Taylor & Francis, London and New York, p. 540.

6 J Semmens, C Tsai and C Loadholt (1985) 'Effects of estrogen therapy on vaginal physiology during menopause', *Obstetrics & Gynecology*, vol. 66, pp. 15–18.

7 GA Bachmann , GA and ID Burd (1999) 'Vulvovaginal complaints' in RA Lobo (ed.) *Treatment of the Postmenopausal Woman: Basic and clinical aspects*, Lippincott Williams & Wilkins, Philadelphia, pp. 195–201; PM Sarrel and B Wiita (1997) 'Vasodilator effects of estrogen are not diminished by androgen in postmenopausal women' *Fertility Sterility*, vol. 68, pp. 1125–7.

8 C Longcope, CC Johnston Jr (1990)'Androgen and estrogen dynamics: stability over a two-year interval in perimenopausal women', *The Journal of Steroid Biochemistry and Molecular Biology*, vol. 35, p. 91; T Lobo (1999) *Treatment of Postmenopausal Women*, Lippincott, Boston.

9 B Zumoff et al (1995) 'Twenty-four hour mean plasma testosterone concentration declines with age in normal premenopausal women', *The Journal of Clinical Endocrinology & Metabolism*; vol. 80, pp. 1429–30; S Davis et al (2002) 'Androgen levels in normal and oophorectomised women' Climacteric, Proceedings of the 10th International Congress on the Menopause, Berlin.

10 JL Shifren (2004) 'The role of androgens in female sexual dysfunction', *Mayo Clinic Proceedings*, vol. 79 (Suppl), pp. S19–S24; JL Shifren et al (2000) 'Transdermal testosterone treatment in women with impaired sexual function after oophorectomy', *The New England Journal of Medicine*, vol. 343, pp. 682–8; SR Davis and HG Burger (1998) 'The rationale for physiological testosterone replacement in women', *Baillière's Clinical Endocrinology and Metabolism*, vol. 12, pp. 391–405.

11 A Traish and N Kim (2006) 'Modulation of female genital sexual arousal by sex steroid hormones' in I Goldstein et al (eds) *Women's Sexual Function and Dysfunction: Study, diagnosis and treatment*, Francis & Taylor, London and New York, p. 187.

12 SR Davis and EA Nijland (2008) 'Pharmacological therapy for female sexual dysfunction: has progress been made?', *Drugs*, vol. 68, no. 3, pp. 259–64; SL Davison et al (2005) 'Androgen levels in adult females: changes with age, menopause, and oophorectomy', *The Journal of Clinical Endocrinology & Metabolism*, vol. 90, no. 7, pp. 3847–53.

13 R Hayes and L Dennerstein (2006) 'Aging issues' in I Goldstein et al (eds) *Women's Sexual Function and Dysfunction: Study, diagnosis and treatment*, Francis & Taylor, London and New York, pp. 245–50.

14 Planned Parenthood of Northern New England, Education Department (2009) 'Week 64: Is it true that men sexually peak at 18 and women around 30?', *Consensual Text*, <http://consensualtext. org/2009/11/week-64-is-it-true-men-sexually-peak-at-18-and-women-around-30/> [accessed 4 March 2010].

15 D Wallechinsky and I Wallace (1975–1981) 'Biography and sexual teachings of Alfred C. Kinsey Part 1', *The People's Almanac*, quoted on <www.trivia-library.com/b/biography-and-sexual-teachings-of-alfred-c-kinsey-part-1.htm> [accessed November 2011].

16 P Shwartz quoted in V Glembocki (2007) 'Paging Mr. December', *Women's Health*, September, p. 98.

17 JD Baldwin and JI Baldwin (1997) 'Gender differences in sexual interest', *Archives of Sexual Behavior*, vol. 26, no. 2, pp. 181–210.

18 DP Schmitt et al (2002) 'Is there an early-30s peak in female sexual desire? Cross-sectional evidence from the United States and Canada', *The Canadian Journal of Human Sexuality*, vol. 11, no. 1, pp. 1–18.

19 M Wiederman (2005) 'The gendered nature of sexual scripts', *The Family Journal: Counseling and Therapy for Couples and Families*, vol. 13, no. 4, pp. 496–502.

20 A Barr, A Bryan and D Kenrick (2002) 'Sexual peak: socially shared cognitions about desire, frequency and satisfaction in men and women', *Personal Relationships*, vol. 9, no. 3, pp. 287–99.

21 D Schnarch (1997) *Passionate Marriage: Keeping love and intimacy alive in committed relationships*, Scribe Publications, Melbourne, p. 76.

22 ibid., p. 78.

23 'Beat your biological clock', *The Independent*, 15 July 2008, <www.independent.co.uk/life-style/health-and-families/healthy-living/beat-your-biological-clock-867508. html?action=Gallery&ino=5> [accessed December 2011].

24 Berman quoted in Glembocki, 'Paging Mr. December', p. 98.

25 J Yadegaran (2008) 'Call older women cougars and some may growl: Other women like predatory moniker', *Ventura County Star*, <www.vcstar.com/news/2008/jul/20/call-them-cougars-and-some-may-growl/ > [accessed 12 March 2010].

26 V Gibson (2002) *Cougar: A guide for older women dating younger men*, Firefly Books, Westport, CT.

27 N Dewolf Smith (2009) *What Women Want (Cont'd)*, *The Wall Street Journal online*, <http://online.wsj.com/article/SB10001424052 9702044883045744432861102779126.html> [accessed April 2010].

28 J Warner (2009) 'The real cougar fans', *New York Times*, <http://opinionator.blogs.nytimes.com/2009/09/24/the-real-cougar-fans/> [accessed 12 March 2010].

Chapter 4

1 F Pittman (1990) *Private Lies: Infidelity and the betrayal of intimacy*, W. W. Norton, New York.

2 MA Whisman et al (2007) 'Predicting sexual infidelity in a population-based sample of married individuals', *Journal of Family Psychology*, vol. 21, no. 2, pp. 320–4.

3 K von Sydow (1999) 'Sexuality during pregnancy and after childbirth: a metacontent analysis of 59 studies', *Journal of Psychosomatic Research*, vol. 47, no. 1, pp. 27–49.

4 M Nash (2007) 'Baby weight-gain scares mums to be', *Today*, <http://today.ninemsn.com.au/healthandbeauty/261739/baby-weight-gain-scares-mums-to-be> [accessed November 2011].

5 I Young (1998) 'Pregnant embodiment' in D Welton (ed.), *Body and Flesh: A philosophical reader*, Blackwell Publishers, p. 279.

6 ibid.

7 ibid.

8 ibid.

9 A Rich (1986) *Of Woman Born: Motherhood as experience and institution*, 10th edn, W.W. Norton & Company, New York, p. 182.

10 ibid., p. 183.

11 S Kitzinger (1983) *Woman's Experience of Sex*, Penguin, Harmondsworth, Middlesex, England.

12 S Mulroy and FJ Stanley (2007) 'Trends in mode of delivery during 1984–2003: can they be explained by pregnancy and delivery complications?', *BJOG: An international journal of obstetrics and gynaecology*, vol. 114, no. 7, pp. 855–64.

13 R Al-Mufti et al (1997) 'Survey of obstetricians' personal preference and discretionary practice', *European Journal of Obstetrics and Gynecology and Reproductive Biology*, vol. 73, no. 1, pp. 1–4.

14 K von Sydow, 'Sexuality during pregnancy and after childbirth', pp. 27–49.

15 Young, 'Pregnant embodiment', p. 280.

16 K von Sydow (2006) 'Pregnancy, childbirth and the postpartum period' in I Goldstein et al (eds) *Women's Sexual Function and Dysfunction: Study, diagnosis and treatment*, Taylor & Francis, London and New York, p. 287.

17 Beyond Blue (2006) 'Types of postnatal depression', <www.beyondblue.org.au/index.aspx?link_id=94.600> [accessed November 2011].

18 Beyond Blue (2009) 'Antenatal and postnatal depression: what puts a person at risk?' <www.beyondblue.org.au/index.aspx?link_id=94.601> [accessed November 2011].

19 SW Chan, V Williamson and H McCutcheon (2009) 'A comparative study of the experiences of a group of Hong Kong Chinese and Australian women diagnosed with Postnatal Depression', *Perspectives in Psychiatric Care*, vol. 45, no. 2, p. 113.

20 ibid., p. 112.

21 A Thompson (2008) 'The rise of the mummy tuck: how new mothers are spending thousands on cosmetic surgery', *MailOnline*, 13 May, <www.dailymail.co.uk/health/article-563799/The-rise-mummy-tuck-How-new-mothers-spending-thousands-cosmetic-surgery.html> [accessed November 2011].

22 A Owens 'Pregnant celebrities "too posh too push"' (2003) *National Post*, 10 February, available at <http://allnurses-central.com/general-off-topic/pregnant-celebrities-too-30944.html> [accessed November 2011].

23 S Kitzinger (1979) *The experience of breastfeeding*, Penguin Books, London, p. 12.

24 S Kitzinger (1983) *Women's experience of sex*, Penguin Books, Harmondsworth, England, p. 45.

25 A Bartlett (2005) *Breastwork: Rethinking breastfeeding*, UNSW Press, Sydney.

26 WH Masters and VE Johnson (1966) *Human Sexual Response*, Little, Brown, Oxford.

27 von Sydow, 'Sexuality during pregnancy and after childbirth', pp. 27–49.

28 F Balsamo et al (1992) 'Production and Pleasure: Research on breast-feeding in Turin', in V Maher (ed.), *The Anthropology of Breast-Feeding*, Oxford, Berg, p. 76.

29 G Greer (1984) *Sex and Destiny: The politics of human fertility*, Harper & Row, New York.

30 L Umansky (1998) 'Breastfeeding in the 1990s: The Karen Carter case and the politics of maternal sexuality', in M Ladd-Taylor and L Umansky (eds), *'Bad' Mothers: The politics of blame in twentieth-century America*, New York University Press, New York.

31 D Fisher (2006) 'Falling in love: the chemistry of the first breastfeed', *Breast is Best*, <www.breast-feeding-information.com/the-chemistry-of-the-first-breastfeed.php> [accessed November 2011].

32 von Sydow, 'Pregnancy, childbirth and the postpartum period', pp. 282–9.

33 Rich, *Of Woman Born*, p. 183.

34 A Waldman (2005) 'Truly, madly, guiltily', *The New York Times*, <www.nytimes.com/2005/03/27/fashion/27love.html> [accessed 27 February 2011].

35 E Perel (2007) *Mating in Captivity: Sex, lies and domestic bliss*, Hodder & Stoughton, London.

36 T Miller (2010) *Making Sense of Fatherhood: Gender, caring and work*, Cambridge University Press, Cambridge.

37 N Oxenhandler (2001) *The Eros of Parenthood: Explorations in light and dark*, St Martin's Press, New York, p. 11.

38 Perel, *Mating in Captivity*, p. 149.

39 LA Kurdek (1999) 'The nature and predictors of the trajectory of change in marital quality for husbands and wives over the first 10

years of marriage', *Developmental Psychology*, vol. 35, pp. 1283–96.

40 H Willen (1996) 'The impact of wish for children and having children on attainment and importance of life values', *Journal of Comparative Family Studies*, vol. 27, pp. 499–518.

41 JM Twenge et al (2003) 'Parenthood and marital satisfaction: A meta-analytic review', *Journal of Marriage and Family*, vol. 65, no. 3, pp. 574–83.

42 Twenge, 'Parenthood and marital satisfaction', p. 581.

43 ibid., p. 580–581.

44 T Ahlborg et al (2000) 'First-time parent's sexual relationships', *Scandinavian Journal of Sexology*, vol. 3, no. 4, pp. 127–39.

45 MF Ehrenberg et al (2001) 'Childcare task division and shared parenting attitudes in dual-earner families with young children', *Family Relations*, vol. 50, no. 2, pp. 143–53.

46 C Kohler-Riessman (1990) *Divorce talk. Women and men make sense of personal relationships*, Rutgers University Press, New Brunswick.

Chapter 5

1 G Greer (1992) *The Change: Women, aging and the menopause*, Alfred A. Knopf, New York.

2 H Cook (2004) *The Long Sexual Revolution: English women, sex, and contraception 1800–1975*, Oxford University Press, New York, p. 167.

3 G Corey (2009) *Theory and practice of counselling and psychotherapy*, eighth edn, Thompson Brooks/Cole, California, p. 61.

4 K Roberts (2006) *Lotus illustrated dictionary of sex*, Lotus Press, New Delhi, p. 9.

5 W Glassman and M Hadad (2004) *Approaches to Psychology*, Open University Press, Maidenhead, England; R Bocock (2002) *Sigmund Freud*, Routledge, London; P Gay (1998) *Freud: A life for our time*, W. W. Norton, New York; A Storr (2001) *Freud: A very short introduction*, Oxford University Press, Oxford.

6 Corey, *Theory and practice of counselling and psychotherapy*, p. 62.

7 Roberts, *Lotus illustrated dictionary of sex*, p. 95.

8   J Mitchell (1974) *Psychoanalysis and Feminism*, Pantheon Books, New York.

9   F Guterl (2002) 'What Freud got right', *Newsweek*, vol. 140, no. 20, <www.newsweek.com/2002/11/10/what-freud-got-right.html> [accessed 25 February 2011].

10 H McFarland Solomon (2003) 'Freud and Jung: an incomplete encounter', *Journal of Analytical Psychology*, vol. 48, p. 554.

11 P Bishop (1999) *Jung in Contexts: A reader*, Routledge, London; S Shamdasani (2003) *Jung and the Making of Modern Psychology: The dream of a science*, Cambridge University Press, Cambridge.

12 C Jung (1956) 'The Concept of Libido' in *Collected works of C.G. Jung*, vol. 5, Routledge, London, pp. 132–41; A Samuels (1986) *Jung and the Post-Jungians*, Routledge, London.

13 E Hoffman (1996) *The Drive for Self: Alfred Adler and the founding of individual psychology*, Addison Wesley, Reading, MA.

14 A Boskovic (1999) 'Lecture 4: Ourselves as others', <www.gape.org/sasa/lecture204.htm> [accessed 27 February 2011].

15 R Saleel (2002) 'Love Anxieties', in S Barnard and B Fink (eds), Reading Seminar XX. *Lacan's Major Work on Love, Knowledge, and Feminine Sexuality*, State University of New York Press, pp. 93–7.

16 M-C Laznik (2005) 'Jouissance (Lacan)', in A de Mijolla (ed.), *International Dictionary of Psychoanalysis*, Gale/Cengage Learning, UK.

17 L Irigaray (1992) *Elemental Passions*, Continuum-Routledge, New York.

18 H Fisher et al (2002) 'Defining the brain systems of lust, romantic attraction and attachment', *Archives of Sexual Behavior*, vol. 31, no. 5, pp. 413–19.

19 B Schaeffer (1999) *Is It Love or Is It Addiction?*, Hazelden, New York, p. 27.

20 D Marazziti et al (1999) 'Alteration of the serotonin transporter in romantic love', *Psychological Medicine*, vol. 29, pp. 741–5.

21 M Lebowitz (1983) *The Chemistry of Love*, Little, Brown, Boston.

22 JG Pfaus (2009) 'Pathways of sexual desire', *Journal of Sexual Medicine*, vol. 6, pp. 1506–33.

23 JG Pfaus et al (2003) 'What can animal models tell us about human sexual response?', *Annual Review of Sex Research*, vol. 14, p. 41.

24 Pfaus, 'Pathways of sexual desire', pp. 1506–33.

25 K Wallen (1995) 'The evolution of female sexual desire', in PR Abramson and SD Pinkerton (eds) *Sexual nature sexual culture*, University of Chicago Press, Chicago, pp. 57–79.

26 BGA Stuckey (2008) 'Female sexual function and dysfunction in the reproductive years: the influence of endogenous and exogenous sex hormones', *Journal of Sexual Medicine*, vol. 5, no. 10, pp. 2282–90.

27 AK Slob et al (1996) 'Sexual arousability and the menstrual cycle', *Psychoneuroendocrinology*, vol. 21, no. 6, pp. 545–58.

28 G Miller et al (2007) 'Ovulatory cycle effects on tip earnings by lap dancers: economic evidence for human estrus?', *Evolution and Human Behavior*, vol. 28, no. 6, pp. 375–81.

29 Pfaus, 'What can animal models tell us about human sexual response?', pp. 1–63.

30 ibid., p. 46.

31 ibid., pp. 19–20.

32 R Basson et al (2003) 'Definitions of women's sexual dysfunction reconsidered: advocating expansion and revision', *Journal of Psychosomatic Obstetrics & Gynecology*, vol. 24, no. 4, pp. 221–9.

33 Pfaus, 'What can animal models tell us about human sexual response?', p. 3.

34 Pfaus, 'Pathways of sexual desire', p. 1507.

35 Pfaus, 'What can animal models tell us about human sexual response?', p. 20.

36 ibid., p. 6.

37 Pfaus, 'Pathways of sexual desire', p. 1513.

38 S Nash and M Domjan (1991) 'Learning to discriminate the sex of conspecifics in male Japanese quail (*Coturnix coturnix japonica*): Tests of "biological constraints"', *Journal of Experimental Psychology: Animal Behavior Processes*, vol. 17, pp. 342–53.

39 Pfaus, 'What can animal models tell us about human sexual response?', p. 42.

40 ibid.

41 ibid., p. 44.

42 Pfaus, 'Pathways of sexual desire', p. 1522.

43   WH Masters and VE Johnson (1966) *Human Sexual Response*, Little, Brown, Boston.

44   C Mantak et al (2000) *The Multi-Orgasmic Couple: Sexual secrets every couple should know*, HarperCollins, New York, p 46

45   L Rosen and R Rosen (2006) 'Fifty years of female sexual dysfunction research and concepts: from Kinsey to the present', in I Goldstein et al (eds) *Sexual Function and Dysfunction: Study, diagnosis and treatment*, Francis & Taylor, London and New York, p. 6.

46   HS Kaplan (1979) *Disorders of Sexual Desire and Other New Concepts and Techniques in Sex Therapy*, Brunner/Hazel Publications, New York.

47   H Lief (1977) 'Inhibited sexual desire', *Medical Aspects of Human Sexuality*, vol. 7, pp. 94–5.

48   B Zilbergeld and C Ellison (1980) 'Desire discrepancies and arousal problems in sexual therapy' in L S and L Pervin (eds), *Principles and Practice of Sex Therapy*, The Guilford Press, New York, pp. 65–101.

49   S Whalen and D Roth (1987) 'A cognitive approach', in J Geer and W O'Donahue (eds), *Theories of Human Sexuality*, Plenum, New York, pp. 335–62.

50   J Bancroft (1983) *Human Sexuality and its Problems*, Churchill Livingstone, New York.

51   WR Stayton and DW Haffner (1998) 'Sexuality and reproductive health in R Hatcher et al (eds) *Contraceptive Technology*, 17th edn, Ardent Media, New York.

52   B Whipple and K Brash-McGreer (1997) 'Management of female sexual dysfunction' in ML Sipski and CJ Alexander (eds) *Sexual Function in People with Disability and Chronic Illness: A health professional's guide*, Aspen Publishers, Gaithersburg, MD, pp. 509–34.

53   MA Perelman (2006) 'A new combination treatment for premature ejaculation: a sex therapist's perspective', *Journal of Sexual Medicine*, vol. 3, pp. 1004–12.

54   C Meston and DM Buss (2009) *Why Women Have Sex: Sexual motivation from adventure to revenge (and everything in between)*, The Bodley Head, London.

55   R Basson (2001) 'Using a different model for female sexual

response to address women's problematic low sexual desire', *Journal of Sex & Marital Therapy*, vol. 27, no. 5, pp. 396–7.

56 R Basson (2000) 'The female sexual response: a different model', *Journal of Sex & Marital Therapy*, vol. 26, no. 1, p. 53.

57 ibid., p. 52.

58 Basson, 'Using a different model for female sexual response', p. 396.

59 ibid., p. 402–3.

60 M Sand and WA Fisher (2007) 'Women's endorsement of models of female sexual response: the nurses' sexuality study', *Journal of Sexual Medicine*, vol. 4, no. 3, pp. 708–19.

61 W Simon and J Gagnon (1986) 'Sexual scripts: performance and change', *Archives of Sexual Behavior*, vol. 15, pp. 97–120.

62 B Ellwood-Clayton (2005) 'Desire and loathing in the cyber Philippines' in R Harper (ed.) *The Inside Text: Social perspectives on SMS in the mobile age*, Springer-Verlag, London, pp. 195–219.

63 B Ellwood-Clayton (2007) 'Constructions of Seduction: Premarital sex in the Catholic Philippines', *Pilipinas*, vol. 46, pp. 1–27.

64 L Manderson and P Liamputtong (2002) *Coming of Age in South and Southeast Asia: Youth, courtship and sexuality*, Routledge/Curzon, London.

65 G Rubin (1984) 'Thinking sex: notes for a radical theory of the politics of sexuality', in C Vance (ed.), *Pleasure and Danger: Exploring female sexuality*, Routledge, Boston, pp. 143–78.

66 J D'Emilio and EB Freedman (1988) *Intimate Matters: A history of sexuality in America*, 2nd edn, The University of Chicago Press, Chicago.

67 G Greer (1970) *The Female Eunuch*, MacGibbon & Kee, London.

68 G Rubin (1984) 'Thinking sex: notes for a radical theory of the politics of sexuality' in C Vance (ed.), *Pleasure and Danger: Exploring female sexuality*, Routledge, New York, pp. 143–78.

69 C Vance (ed.), *Pleasure and Danger: Exploring female sexuality*, Routledge, Boston.

Chapter 6

1 G Hart and K Wellings (2002) 'Sexual behaviour and its medicalisation: in sickness and in health', *British Medical Journal*, vol. 324, p. 896.

2   R Moynihan (2005) 'The marketing of a disease: female sexual dysfunction', *British Medical Journal*, vol. 330, p. 192.

3   ibid., p. 192.

4   ibid., p. 194.

5   Goodman, '"Why not me?"', <http://inventorspot.com/articles/fda_turns_down_drug_called_female_viagra_43700>.

6   EO Laumann, A Paik and RC Rosen (1999) 'Sexual dysfunction in the United States: prevalence and predictors', *JAMA*, vol. 281, pp. 537–44.

7   L Tiefer (2001) 'A new view of women's sexual problems: Why new? Why now?', *The Journal of Sex Research*, vol. 38, no. 2, pp. 89–96.

8   M King et al (2007) 'Women's views of their sexual difficulties: agreement and disagreement with clinical diagnoses', *Archives of Sexual Behavior*, vol. 36, pp. 281–8.

9   ibid., p. 287.

10   ibid., p. 281.

11   U Hartmann et al (2002) 'Female sexual desire disorders: subtypes, classification, personality factors and new directions for treatment', *World Journal of Urology*, vol. 20, pp. 79–88.

12   M Foucault (1979) *Discipline and Punish: The birth of the prison*, Vintage, New York.

13   B Deer (2003) 'Love sickness', *The Sunday Times Magazine*, 28 September, p. 4.

14   L Tiefer (2006) 'Female sexual dysfunction: a case study of disease mongering and activist resistance', *Plos Medicine*, vol. 3, no. 4, pp. 36–40.

15   R Moynihan (2003) 'The making of a disease: female sexual dysfunction', *British Medical Journal*, vol. 326, p. 45.

16   American Psychiatric Association (2000) *Diagnostic and Statistical Manual of Mental Disorders*, 4th edn.

17   J Berman et al (2001) *For Women Only: A revolutionary guide to reclaiming your sex life*, Henry Holt & Co., New York.

18   L Dennerstein et al (2006) 'Hypoactive Sexual Desire Disorder in menopausal women: a survey of Western European women', *Journal of Sexual Medicine*, vol. 3, pp. 212–22.

19   G Bachmann (2006) 'Female sexuality and sexual dysfunction: are

we stuck on the learning curve?', *Journal of Sexual Medicine*, vol. 3, pp. 639–45.

20 G Brock et al (2002) 'Sexual problems in mature men and women: results of a global study', *International Journal of Impotence Research*, vol. 13, no. 3 (supplementary), pp. S57–8.

21 RD Hayes et al (2008) 'What is the "true" prevalence of Female Sexual Dysfunction and does the way we assess these conditions have an impact?', *Journal of Sexual Medicine*, vol. 5, pp. 777–87.

22 ibid., p. 784.

23 AH Clayton et al (2009) 'Validation of the decreased sexual desire screener (DSDS): a brief diagnostic instrument for generalized acquired female Hypoactive Sexual Desire Disorder (HSDD)', *Journal of Sexual Medicine*, vol. 6, pp. 730–8.

24 YR Avellanet et al (2008) 'Relationship between loss of libido and signs and symptoms of depression in a sample of Puerto Rican middle-aged women', *Puerto Rico Health Sciences Journal*, vol. 27, no. 1, pp. 85–91.

25 Sl West et al (2008) 'Prevalence of low sexual desire and hypoactive sexual desire disorder in a nationally representative sample of US women', *Archives of Internal Medicine*, vol. 168, no. 13, pp. 1441–9.

26 J Richters et al (2003) 'Sex in Australia: sexual difficulties in a representative sample of adults', *Australian and New Zealand Journal of Public Health*, vol. 27, no. 2, pp. 164–70.

27 RD Hayes et al (2008) 'Risk factors for Female Sexual Dysfunction in the general population: exploring factors associated with low sexual function and sexual distress', *Journal of Sexual Medicine*, vol. 5, no. 7, pp. 1681–93.

28 ibid., p.1681.

29 A Nicolosi et al (2005) 'Sexual behaviour and dysfunction and help-seeking patterns in adults aged 40–80 years in the urban population of Asian countries', *BJU International*, vol. 95, pp. 609–14.

30 ED Moreira Jr et al (2005) 'Sexual activity, sexual dysfunction and associated help-seeking behaviours in middle-aged and older adults in Spain: a population survey', *World Journal of Urology*, vol. 23, pp. 422–9.

31 Avellanet, 'Relationship between loss of libido and signs and symptoms of depression', p. 88.

32 Richters, 'Sex in Australia', pp. 164–70.

33 ibid.

34 LA Brotto (2009) 'The DSM diagnostic criteria for Hypoactive Sexual Desire Disorder in women', *Archives of Sexual Behavior*.

35 MA Perelman (2006) 'A new combination treatment for premature ejaculation: a sex therapist's perspective', *Journal of Sexual Medicine*, vol. 3, pp. 1004–12.

36 LH Clarke (2006) 'Older women and sexuality: experiences in marital relationships across the life course', *Canadian Journal on Aging*, vol. 25, no. 2, pp. 129–40.

Chapter 7

1 J Kenyon, 'Back', *The New Yorker*, 23 September 1991.

2 'Depression', World Health Organization, <www.who.int/mental_health/management/depression/definition/en/> [accessed October 2010].

3. SJ Bunker et al (2003) '"Stress" and coronary heart disease: psychosocial risk factors', *The Medical Journal of Australia*, vol. 178, no. 6, pp. 272–6.

4 'Women and depression' (2008) National Institute of Mental Health, <www.nimh.nih.gov/health/publications/depression/the-numbers-count-mental-disorders-in-america/index.shtml> [accessed 21 May 2009].

5 D Rose (2007) 'Britain becomes a Prozac nation', *The Times*, <www.dailymail.co.uk/health/article-454678/Doctors-hand-record-31m-anti-depressant-prescriptions.html> [accessed 20 May 2009]

6 American Psychiatric Association (2000) *Diagnostic and Statistical Manual of Mental Disorders*, 4th edn.

7 ibid.

8 RC Kessler et al (2003) 'The epidemiology of major depressive disorder results from the National Comorbidity Survey Replication (NCS-R)', *JAMA*, vol. 289, no. 23, pp. 3095–105.

9 'Depression & Women' (2006) National Women's Health Report, vol. 25, no. 4.

10 National Institute of Mental Health (2008) 'Women and

depression', <www.nimh.nih.gov/health/publications/depression/the-numbers-count-mental-disorders-in-america/index.shtml> [accessed 21 May 2009].

11 ibid.

12 Australian Bureau of Statistics (2008) 'How Australians use their time, 2006', <www.abs.gov.au/AUSSTATS/abs@.nsf/Latestproducts/4153.0Main%20Features22006?opendocument&tabname=Summary&prodno=4153.0&issue=2006&num=&view=> [accessed February 2011].

13 PE Bebbington (1998) 'Editorial: sex and depression', *Psychological Medicine*, vol. 28, no. 1, pp. 1–8.

14 CM Mazure and PK Maciejewski (2003) 'The interplay of stress, gender and cognitive style in depressive onset', *Archive of Women's Mental Health*, vol. 6, pp. 5–8.

15 KS Kendler et al (2001) 'Gender differences in the rates of exposure to stressful life events and sensitivity to their depressogenic effects', *American Journal of Psychiatry*, vol. 158, no. 4, pp. 587–93.

16 RJ Turner and WR Avison (1989) 'Gender and depression: assessing exposure and vulnerability to life events in a chronically strained population', *Journal of Nervous and Mental Disease*, vol. 177, pp. 443–55.

17 P Kramer (2005) *Against Depression*, Viking Adult, New York.

18 B McLellan (1995) *Beyond Psychoppression: A feminist alternative therapy*, Spinefex Press, North Melbourne, p. 34.

19 U Werneke et al (2006) 'Antidepressants and sexual dysfunction', *Acta Psychiatrica Scandinavica*, vol. 114, p. 392.

20 RL Phillips and JR Slaughter (2000) 'Depression and sexual desire', *American Family Physician*, vol. 62, pp. 782–6.

21 JM Cyranowski et al (2004) 'Lifetime depression history and sexual function in women at midlife', *Archives of Sexual Behavior*, vol. 33, no. 6, pp. 539–49.

22 A Deeks (2008) *Low Libido: The psychological aspect*, <www.menopause.org.au/health-professionals/gp-a-hp-resources/195> [accessed 24 February 2011].

23 K Williams and MF Reynolds (2006) 'Sexual dysfunction in major depression', *CNS Spectrums*, vol. 11, pp. 19–23; RL Phillips and

JR Slaughter (2000) 'Depression and sexual desire', *American Family Physician*, vol. 62, pp. 782–6.

24 P Hensley and G Nurnberg (2006) 'Depression' in MZ Goldstein et al (eds), *Women's Sexual Function and Dysfunction: Study, diagnosis and treatment*, Taylor & Francis, London and New York, p. 619.

25 YR Avellanet et al (2008) 'Relationship between loss of libido and signs and symptoms of depression in a sample of Puerto Rican middle-aged women', *Puerto Rico Health Sciences Journal*, vol. 27, no. 1, p. 86.

26 Wurtzel, E 1994, *Prozac Nation: Young and depressed in America*, Houghton Mifflin, Boston.

27 McLellan, *Beyond Psychoppression*, p. 34.

28 D Woodlock (2005) 'Virtual pushers: antidepressant internet marketing and women', *Women's Studies International Forum*, vol. 28, no. 4, p. 306.

29 SD Hollon et al (2003) 'Treatment and prevention of depression', *Psychological Science in the Public Interest*, vol. 2, no. 2, pp. 39–70.

30 'Depression', World Health Organization, <www.who.int/mental_health/management/depression/definition/en/> [accessed October 2010].

31 AH Clayton (2002) 'Female sexual dysfunction related to depression and antidepressant medications', *Current Women's Health Reports*, no. 2, pp. 182–7.

32 'Prozac makes history' (2011) <www.prozac.com/Pages/index.aspx> [accessed March 2009].

33 G Nurnberg et al (2008) 'Sildenafil treatment of women with antidepressant-associated sexual dysfunction: a randomized controlled trial', *JAMA*, vol. 300, no. 4, pp. 395–404.

34 D Woodlock (2005) 'Virtual pushers: antidepressant internet marketing and women', *Women's Studies International Forum*, vol. 28, no. 4, p. 305.

35 ibid., p. 305.

36 U Lovdahl et al (1999) 'Gender display in Scandinavian and American advertising for antidepressants', *Scandinavian Journal of Public Health*, vol. 27, pp. 306–10.

37   U Werneke et al (2006) 'Antidepressants and sexual dysfunction',
     Acta Psychiatrica Scandinavica, vol. 114, p. 385.

38   G Nurnberg et al (2008) 'Sildenafil treatment of women with anti-
     depressant-associated sexual dysfunction: a randomized controlled
     trial', *JAMA*, vol. 300, no. 4, pp. 395–404.

39   P Hensley and G Nurnberg (2006) 'Depression' in MZ Goldstein
     et al (eds), *Women's Sexual Function and Dysfunction: Study,
     diagnosis and treatment*, Taylor & Francis, London and New
     York, p. 619.

40   LA Piazza et al (1997) 'Sexual functioning in chronically depressed
     patients treated with SSRI antidepressants: A pilot study', *Amer-
     ican Journal of Psychiatry*, vol. 154, no. 12, pp. 1757–9.

41   Al Montejo et al (2001) 'Incidence of sexual dysfunction associ-
     ated with antidepressant agents: a prospective multicenter study of
     1022 outpatients', *Journal of Clinical Psychiatry*, vol. 62, no.
     suppl 3, pp. 10–21; AL Montejo-Gonzalez et al (1997) 'SSRI-
     induced sexual dysfunction: fluoxetine, paroxetine, sertaline, and
     fluvoxamine in a prospective, multicenter, and descriptive clinical
     study of 344 patients', *Journal of Sex & Marital Therapy*, vol. 23,
     pp. 176–94.

42   JM Cyranowski et al (2004) 'Lifetime depression history and
     sexual function in women at midlife', *Archives of Sexual Behavior*,
     vol. 33, no. 6, pp. 539–49.

43   Werneke, 'Antidepressants and sexual dysfunction', pp. 384–97.

44   HE Fisher and JA Thomson (2006) 'Lust, romance, attachment:
     do the sexual side effects of serotonin-enhancing antidepressants
     jeopardize romantic love, marriage, and fertility?' in S Platek, J
     Keenan and T Shackelford (eds), *Evolutionary Cognitive Neuro-
     science*, The MIT Press, Cambridge, pp. 245–83.

45   AJ Mitchell and T Selmes (2007) 'Why don't patients take their
     medicine? Reasons and solutions in psychiatry', *Advances in
     Psychiatric Treatment*, vol. 13, no. 5, pp. 336–46.

46   A Rothschild (1995) 'Selective serotonin reuptake inhibitor-
     induced sexual dysfunction: efficacy of a drug holiday', *The
     American Journal of Psychiatry*, vol. 152, pp. 1514–6.

47   Hensley and Nurnberg, 'Depression' in Goldstein et al, *Women's
     Sexual Function and Dysfunction*, p. 622.

48 JM Ferguson (2001) 'The effects of antidepressants on sexual functioning in depressed patients: a review', *Journal of Clinical Psychiatry*, vol. 62, supp. 3, pp. 22–34.

49 A Clayton et al (2004) 'A placebo-controlled trial of bupropion SR as an antidote for selective serotonin reuptake inhibitor-induced sexual dysfunction', *Journal of Clinical Psychiatry*, vol. 65, no. 1, pp. 62–7.

50 RC Rosen, RM Lane and M Menza (1999) 'Effects of SSRIs on sexual function: a critical review', *Journal of Clinical Psychopharmacology*, vol. 1967, pp. 67–85.

51 N Schimelpfening (2011) 'Antidepressants and Sexual Dysfunction: Tips to reduce sexual side effects', <http://depression.about.com/od/sexualdysfunction/a/sexdysfunction.htm> [accessed September 2011].

52 G Nurnberg et al (2008) 'Sildenafil treatment of women with anti-depressant-associated sexual dysfunction: a randomized controlled trial', *JAMA*, vol. 300, no. 4, pp. 395–404.

53 Hensley and Nurnberg, 'Depression' in Goldstein et al, *Women's Sexual Function and Dysfunction*, pp. 622–3.

54 A Rothschild (1995) 'Selective serotonin reuptake inhibitor-induced sexual dysfunction: efficacy of a drug holiday', *American Journal of Psychiatry*, vol. 152, pp. 1514–16.

55 Hensley and Nurnberg, 'Depression' in Goldstein et al, *Women's Sexual Function and Dysfunction*, p. 622.

Chapter 8

1 'A Profile of Older Americans: 2010' (2010) Administration on Aging, U.S. Department of Health and Human Services, <www.aoa.gov/aoaroot/aging_statistics/Profile/2010/docs/2010profile.pdf>.

2 O Kontula and A Miettinen (2005) *Synthesis report on demographic behaviour, existing population related policies and expectations men and women have concerning the state*, The Population Research Institute, Family Federation of Finland, DIALOG Work package 4, Report D15, Helsinki.

3 N Warren (2007) *Markers of Midlife: Interrogating health, illness and ageing in rural Australia*, The University of Melbourne.

4   P Laslett (1991) *A Fresh Map of Life: The emergence of the Third Age*, Weidenfeld & Nicholson, London.

5   M Featherstone and M Hepworth (1991) 'The mask of ageing and the postmodern life course' in M Featherstone et al (eds) *The Body: Social process and cultural theory*, Sage, London, pp. 371–89.

6   BS Turner (1995) 'Aging and identity: some reflections on the somatization of the self' in M Featherstone and A Wernick (eds) *Images of Aging: Cultural representations of later life*, Routledge, London, pp. 245–60; K Ballard et al (2005) 'Beyond the mask: women's experiences of public and private ageing during midlife and their use of age-resisting activities', *Health*, vol. 9, no. 2, pp. 169–87.

7   RC Atchley (1989) 'A continuity theory of normal aging', *The Gerontologist*, vol. 29, no. 2, pp. 183–90.

8   SR Sherman (1994) 'Changes in age identity: self-perceptions in middle and late-life', *Journal of Aging Studies*, vol. 8, no. 4, pp. 397–412.

9   AE Barrett (2003) 'Socioeconomic status and age identity: The role of dimensions of health in the subjective construction of age', *The Journals of Gerontology*, vol. 58B, no. 2, pp. S101–S9.

10 K Ballard et al (2001) 'The role of the menopause in women's experiences of the "change of life"', *Sociology of Health & Illness*, vol. 23, no. 4, pp. 397–424.

11 M Hepworth (2000) *Stories of Ageing*, Open University Press, Buckingham.

12 EM Astbury-Ward (2003) 'Menopause, sexuality and culture: is there a universal experience?', *Sexual and Relationship Therapy*, vol. 18, no. 4, pp. 437–45; Ballard, 'The role of the menopause in women's experiences', pp. 397–424.

13 Astbury-Ward, 'Menopause, sexuality and culture', pp. 437–45.

14 P Oberg and L Tornstam (1999) 'Body images among men and women of different ages', *Ageing & Society*, vol. 19, pp. 629–44.

15 S Sontag (1978) 'The double standard of ageing' in V Carver and P Liddiard (eds) *An Ageing Population: A reader and sourcebook*, Hodder & Stoughton in association with Open University Press, Seven Oaks, pp. 72–80.

16 P Oberg and L Tornstam (1999) 'Body images among men and women of different ages', *Ageing & Society*, vol. 19, pp. 629–44.

17 EM Astbury-Ward (2003) 'Menopause, sexuality and culture: is there a universal experience?', *Sexual and Relationship Therapy*, vol. 18, no. 4, pp. 437–45.

18 Warren, *Markers of Midlife*.

19 O Kontula and A Miettinen (2005) *Synthesis report on demographic behaviour, existing population related policies and expectations men and women have concerning the state*, The Population Research Institute, Family Federation of Finland, DIALOG Work package 4, Report D15, Helsinki.

20 JC Rhodes, KH Kjerulff and PW Langenberg (1999) 'Hysterectomy and sexual functioning', *JAMA*, vol. 282, p. 1934.

21 B Zumoff et al (1995) 'Twenty four hour mean plasma testosterone concentration declines with age in normal premenopausal women', *The Journal of Clinical Endocrinology & Metabolism*, vol. 80, pp. 1429–30.

22 SL Davison et al (2005) 'Androgen levels in adult females: changes with age, menopause, and oophorectomy', *The Journal of Clinical Endocrinology & Metabolism*, vol. 90, no. 7, pp. 3847–53; H Burger, E Dudley and J Cui (2000) 'A prospective longitudinal study of serum testosterone, dehydroepiandrosterone sulfate, and sex-hormone binding globulin levels though the menopausal transition', *Journal of Clinical Endocrinology & Metabolism*, vol. 85, no. 8, pp. 2832–8.

23 A Altman and D Deldon-Saltin (2006) 'Available therapies and outcome results in transition and postmenopausal women' in I Goldstein et al (eds) *Women's Sexual Function and Dysfunction: Study, diagnosis and treatment*, Taylor & Francis, London and New York, pp. 549–59.

24 SA Kingsberg (2002) 'The impact of aging on sexual function in women and their partners', *Archives of Sexual Behavior*, vol. 31, no. 5, p. 433.

25 L Dennerstein et al (2004) 'A population-based study of depressed mood in middle-aged Australian-born women', *Menopause*, vol. 11, pp. 563–8.

26 E Freeman (2010) 'Associations of depression with the transition to menopause', *Menopause*, vol. 17, no. 4, p. 823.

27 PA Kaufert et al (1987) 'Defining menopausal status: the impact of longitudinal data', *Maturitas*, vol. 9, no. 3, pp. 217–26.

28 M Lock (1998) 'Menopause: lessons from anthropology', *Psychosomatic Medicine*, vol. 60, no. 4, pp. 410–19.

29 P Kaufert (1982) 'Anthropology and the menopause: the development of a theoretical framework', *Maturitas*, vol. 4, pp. 181–93.

30 Y Beyene (1986) 'Cultural significance and physiological manifestations of menopause: a biocultural analysis', *Culture, Medicine and Psychiatry*, vol. 10, pp. 47–71.

31 'New research on menopause and sexuality finds women are not seeking medical help for chronic symptoms affecting intimate relationships', 2001, *PR Newswire* <www.prnewswire.com/news-releases/new-research-on-menopause-and-sexuality-finds-women-are-not-seeking-medical-help-for-chronic-symptoms-affecting-intimate-relationships-74273812.html> [accessed 25 February 2011].

32 GE Berger (1999) *Menopause and Culture*, Pluto, London.

33 N Warren (2007) 'Markers of midlife: interrogating health, illness and ageing in rural Australia', The University of Melbourne.

34 E Freeman et al (2007) 'Symptoms associated with menopausal transition and reproductive hormones in midlife women', *Obstetrics & Gynecology*, vol. 110, no. 2, pp. 230–40.

35 E Freeman (2010) 'Associations of depression with the transition to menopause', *Menopause*, vol. 17, no. 4, p. 823.

36 JEM Blumel et al (2004) 'Relationship between psychological complaints and vasomotor symptoms during climacteric', *Maturitas*, vol. 49, no. 3, pp. 205–10.

37 P Love and J Robinson (1994) *Hot Monogamy: Essential steps to more passionate, intimate lovemaking*, Dutton, New York, p. 371.

38 DC Dugdale III (2010) 'Aging changes in the senses', *MedlinePlus*, <www.nlm.nih.gov/medlineplus/ency/article/004013.htm> [accessed January 2011].

39 A Huang et al (2009) 'Sexual function and aging in racially and ethnically diverse women', *The Journal of the American Geriatrics Society*, vol. 57, pp. 1362–8.

40 RD Hayes and L Dennerstein (2005) 'The impact of aging on sexual function and sexual dysfunction in women: a review of population-based studies', *Journal of Sex Medicine*, vol. 2,

pp. 317–30; ST Lindau et al (2007) 'A study of sexuality and health among older adults in the United States', *The New England Journal of Medicine*, vol. 23, pp. 762–4; A Nicolosi et al (2006) 'Sexual behaviour, sexual dysfunctions and related help seeking patterns in middle-aged and elderly Europeans: The global study of sexual attitudes and behaviors', *World Journal of Urology*, vol. 24, pp. 423–8.

41 Huang, 'Sexual function and aging in racially and ethnically diverse women', pp. 1362–8.

42 Lindau et al, 'A study of sexuality and health among older adults in the United States', pp. 762–4.

43 B Bartlik and MZ Goldstein (2001) 'Men's sexual health after midlife', *Psychiatric Services*, vol. 52, no. 3, pp. 291–306.

44 NE Avis et al (2009) 'Longitudinal changes in sexual functioning as women transition through menopause: results from the Study of Women's Health Across the Nation', *Menopause*, vol. 16, no. 3, pp. 442–52; Huang, 'Sexual function and aging in racially and ethnically diverse women', pp. 1362–8.

45 U Hartmann et al (2004) 'Low sexual desire in midlife and older women: personality factors, psychosocial development, present sexuality', *Menopause*, vol. 11, pp. 726–40.

46 JD DeLamater and M Sil (2005) 'Sexual desire in later life', *Journal of Sex Research*, vol. 42, pp. 138–49.

47 ibid.

48 LM Carpenter, CA Nathanson and YJ Kim (2009) 'Physical women, emotional men; gender and sexual satisfaction in midlife', *Archives of Sexual Behavior*, vol. 38, no. 1, pp. 87–107.

49 L Dennerstein, P Lehert and H Burger (2005) 'The relative effects of hormones and relationship factors on sexual function of women through natural menopause transition', *Fertility and Sterility*, vol. 84, pp. 174–80.

50 L Manderson (2005) 'The social and cultural context of sexual function among middle-aged women', *Menopause*, vol. 12, no. 4, pp. 361–2.

51 Huang, 'Sexual function and aging in racially and ethnically diverse women', p. 1362.

52 ibid., pp. 1362–8.

53 NE Avis et al (2009) 'Longitudinal changes in sexual functioning as women transition through menopause: results from the Study of Women's Health Across the Nation', *Menopause*, vol. 16, no. 3, p. 451.

54 L Croft (1982) *Sexuality in Later Life: A counseling guide for physicians*, PSG Inc, Boston.

55 G Trudel, L Turgeon and L Piche (2000) 'Marital and sexual aspects of old age', *Sexual and Relationship Therapy*, vol. 15, pp. 381–406.

56 J DeLamater and SM Moorman (2007) 'Sexual behavior in later life', *Journal of Aging and Health*, vol. 19, no. 6, pp. 921–45.

57 DeLamater and Sil, 'Sexual desire in later life', pp. 138–49.

58 W Masters, V Johnson and R Kolodny (1994) *Heterosexuality*, Harper Collins, New York.

59 The National Council on Aging (1998) 'Healthy sexuality and vital aging', <www.cin-ncoa.org/love/natural_part.htm> [accessed September 2010].

60 LH Clarke (2006) 'Older women and sexuality: experiences in marital relationships across the life course', *Canadian Journal on Aging*, vol. 25, no. 2, pp. 129–40.

61 'Old-age "tsar" promotes sex' (2001) *BBC News* <http://news.bbc. co.uk/2/hi/health/1541706.stm> [accessed 22 June 2010].

62 Avis et al, 'Longitudinal changes in sexual functioning as women transition through menopause', p. 442.

63 ibid.

64 M Patel, C Brown and G Bachmann (2006) 'Sexual function in the menopause and perimenopause ' in I Goldstein et al (eds) *Women's Sexual Function and Dysfunction*, Taylor & Francis, London and New York, pp. 251–62; L Dennerstein and I Goldstein (2005) 'Postmenopausal female sexual dysfunction: at a crossroads', *Journal of Sex Medicine*, vol. 2, pp. 116–17.

65 Avis et al, 'Longitudinal changes in sexual functioning as women transition through menopause', p. 442.

66 L Dennerstein, E Dudley and H Burger (2001) 'Are changes in sexual functioning during midlife due to aging or menopause?', *Fertility and Sterility*, vol. 76, pp. 456–60.

67 CR Gracia et al (2007) 'Hormones and sexuality during transition to menopause', *Obstetrics & Gynecology*, vol. 109, pp. 831–40.

68 Hayes and Dennerstein, 'The impact of aging on sexual function and sexual dysfunction in women', pp. 317–30.

69 C Gracia et al (2004) 'Predictors of decreased libido in women during the late reproductive years', *Menopause*, vol. 11, no. 2, p. 149.

70 Gracia et al, 'Hormones and sexuality during transition to menopause', p. 837.

71 Gracia et al, 'Predictors of decreased libido in women during the late reproductive years', p. 147.

72 L Dennerstein et al (2008) 'Sexual function, dysfunction, and sexual distress in a prospective, population-based sample of mid-aged, Australian-born women', *Journal of Sexual Medicine*, vol. 5, pp. 2291–9.

73 L Dennerstein et al (2006) 'Hypoactive Sexual Desire Disorder in menopausal women: a survey of Western European women', *Journal of Sexual Medicine*, vol. 3, p. 213.

74 SA Kingsberg (2002) 'The impact of aging on sexual function in women and their partners', *Archives of Sexual Behavior*, vol. 31, no. 5, p. 436.

75 ibid.

76 JA Winterich (2003) 'Sex, menopause, and culture: sexual orientation and the meaning of menopause for women's sex lives', *Gender & Society*, vol. 17, no. 4, pp. 627–42.

77 W Dumaresq, personal communication. See also W Dumaresq (2009) *Radiant Women: Simple steps to better menstruation and menopause*, 2nd edn, Natural Woman Network Publication, Mt Clear.

Chapter 9

1 DC Radley et al (2006) 'Off-label prescribing among office-based physicians', *Archives of Internal Medicine*, vol. 166, pp. 1021–6.

2 C Adams (2009) 'Late move on drugs by Bush FDA could be dangerous', *McClatchy*, <www.mcclatchydc.com/2009/02/01/61113/late-move-on-drugs-by-bush-fda.html> [accessed November 2011].

3 R Moynihan (2010) *Sex, Lies and Pharmaceuticals: How drug companies are bankrolling the next big condition for women*, Allen & Unwin, Sydney.

4 JR Berman and L Berman (2001) 'Effect of sildenafil on subjective and physiologic parameters of the female sexual response in women with sexual arousal disorder', *Journal of Sex & Marital Therapy*, vol. 27, pp. 411–20; JR Berman et al (2003) 'Safety and efficacy of sildenafil citrate for the treatment of female sexual arousal disorder: a double-blind, placebo-controlled study', *Journal of Urology*, vol. 170, no. 6, Pt 1, pp. 2333–8; E Laan et al (2002) 'The enhancement of vaginal vasocongestion by sildenafil in healthy premenopausal women', *Journal of Women's Health & Gender-Based Medicine*, vol. 11, pp. 357–65.

5 G Nurnberg et al (2008) 'Sildenafil treatment of women with anti-depressant-associated sexual dysfunction: a randomized controlled trial', *JAMA*, vol. 300, no. 4, pp. 395–404.

6 D Brown, J Kyle and M Ferril (2009) 'Assessing the clinical efficacy of sildenafil for the treatment of female sexual dysfunction', *The Annals of Pharmacotherapy*, vol. 43, no. 7, pp. 1275–85.

7 A O'Connor (2005) 'Dr Berman's sex R$_X$', *Los Angeles Times*, 2 October, <http://articles.latimes.com/2005/oct/02/magazine/tm-sexresearch40> [accessed September 2011].

8 J Block (2011) 'Warning: Orgasm, Inc. will leave you hot and bothered', *Time U.S.*, 11 February <www.time.com/time/nation/article/0,8599,2048609,00.html> [accessed May 2011].

9 R Basson and L Brotto (2003) 'Sexual psychophysiology and effects of sildenafil citrate in oestrogenised women with acquired genital arousal disorder and impaired orgasm: a randomised controlled trial', *BJPG*, vol. 110, pp. 1014–24.

10 SR Davis and EA Nijland (2008) 'Pharmacological therapy for female sexual dysfunction: has progress been made?', *Drugs*, vol. 68, no. 3, pp. 259–64.

11 E Barrett-Connor and CA Stuenkel (2001) 'Hormone replacement therapy (HRT): risks and benefits', *International Journal of Epidemiology*, vol. 30, no. 3, pp. 423–6; J Rymer and EP Morris (2000) 'Menopausal symptoms: extracts from "Clinical Evidence"', *British Medical Journal*, vol. 321, no. 7275, pp. 1516–19; HD Nelson (2004) 'Commonly used types of postmenopausal estrogen for treatment of hot flashes: scientific review', *JAMA*, vol. 291, no. 13, pp. 1610–20.

12 L Dennerstein et al (2006) 'Hypoactive Sexual Desire Disorder in menopausal women: a survey of Western European women', *Journal of Sexual Medicine*, vol. 3, pp. 212–22.

13 PR Casson et al (1997) 'Effect of postmenopausal estrogen replacement on circulating androgens', *Obstetrics & Gynecology*, vol. 90, no. 6, pp. 995–8.

14 A Guay and S Davis (2002) 'Testosterone insufficiency in women: fact or fiction?', *World Journal of Urology*, vol. 20, pp. 106–10; RA Lobo, RC Rosen, H Yang, B Block and RG van der Hoop (2003) 'Comparative effects of oral esterified estrogens with and without methyltestosterone on endocrine profiles and dimensions of sexual function in postmenopausal women with hypoactive sexual desire', *Fertility and Sterility*, vol. 79, no. 6, pp. 1341–52; JL Shifren (2002) 'Androgen deficiency in the oophorectomized woman', *Fertility and Sterility*, vol. 77, suppl., pp. 60–2.

15 RA Wilson (1966) *Feminine Forever*, Lippincott, New York.

16 S Coney (1991) *The Menopause Industry: A guide to medicine's 'discovery' of the mid-life woman*, Penguin Books, Auckland, p. 159.

17 JE Rossouw et al (2002) 'Risks and benefits of estrogen plus progestin in healthy postmenopausal women: principal results from the women's health initiative randomized controlled trial', *JAMA*, vol. 288, no. 3, pp. 321–33.

18 G Anderson et al (2004) 'Effects of conjugated equine estrogen in postmenopausal women with hysterectomy: the Women's Health Initiative randomized controlled trial', *JAMA*, vol. 291, no. 14, pp. 1701–12.

19 E Jungheim and G Colditz (2011) 'Short-term use of unopposed estrogen: A balance of inferred risks and benefits', *JAMA*, vol. 305, no. 13, pp. 1354–5; A LaCroix et al (2011) 'Health outcomes after stopping conjugated equine estrogens among post-menopausal women with prior hysterectomy: A randomized controlled trial', *JAMA*, vol. 305, pp. 1305–14.

20 JE Rossouw et al (2002) 'Risks and benefits of estrogen plus progestin in healthy postmenopausal women: principal results from the women's health initiative randomized controlled trial', *JAMA*, vol. 288, no. 3, pp. 321–33; RT Chlebowski et al (2003) 'Influence of estrogen plus progestin on breast cancer and

mammography in healthy postmenopausal women: the Women's Health Initiative randomized trial', *JAMA*, vol. 289, no. 24, pp. 3243–53.

21 The Women's Health Initiative, participant website (2011) 'Frequently asked questions about estrogen plus progestin and breast cancer' <www.whi.org/faq/faq_bc.php> [accessed November 2011].

22 M Singer (2010) 'Warning of dangers to children, pets from menopause relief spray', *The Age*, 10 August, p. 2.

23 S Somers (2004) *The Sexy Years: Discover the hormone connection. The secret to fabulous sex, great health, and vitality, for women and men*, Crown, New York.

24 R McGraw (2008) *What's Age Got To Do With It? Living your happiest and healthiest life*, Thomas Nelson, Tennessee, p. 117.

25 P Hall, The Oprah Winfrey Show (2009) 'The Great Debate: Should you replace your hormones?', aired 15 January, <www.oprah.com/showinfo/The-Great-Debate-Should-You-Replace-Your-Hormones_1> [accessed November 2011].

26 McGraw, *What's Age Got To Do With It?*, p. 123.

27 C Northrup (2001) *The Wisdom of Menopause: Creating physical and emotional health and healing during the change*, Bantam Dell, New York, pp. 137–8.

28 The Oprah Winfrey Show (2009) 'The Great Debate: Should you replace your hormones?', aired 15 January, <www.oprah.com/showinfo/The-Great-Debate-Should-You-Replace-Your-Hormones_1> [accessed November 2011]; for more of Utian's work see WH Utian et al (2010) 'Estrogen and progestogen use in postmenopausal women: 2010 position statement of The North American Menopause Society', *Menopause*, vol. 17, issue 2, pp. 242–55.

29 Northrup, *The Wisdom of Menopause*, p. 140.

30 S Davis and HG Burger (1999) 'Androgen replacement in women', in AW Meikle (ed.), *Hormone Replacement Therapy*, Humana Press, New Jersey, pp. 401–18.

31 H Burger and M Papalia (2006) 'A clinical update on female androgen insufficiency—testosterone testing and treatment in women presenting with low sexual desire', *Sexual Health*, vol. 3, pp. 73–8.

32 S Bhasin (2005) 'Female Androgen Deficiency Syndrome: an unproven hypothesis', *The Journal of Clinical Endocrinology & Metabolism*, vol. 90, no. 8, pp. 4970–2.

33 SL Davison et al (2005) 'Androgen levels in adult females; changes with age, menopause, and oophorectomy', *The Journal of Clinical Endocrinology & Metabolism*, vol. 90, no. 7, pp. 3847–53.

34 S Bhasin and JG Buckwalter (2001) 'Testosterone supplementation in older men: a rational idea whose time has not yet come', *Journal of Andrology*, vol. 22, issue 5, pp. 718–31.

35 K Miller et al (2006) 'Effects of testosterone replacement in androgen-deficient women with hypopituitarism: a randomized, double-blind, placebo-controlled study', *The Journal of Clinical Endocrinology & Metabolism*, vol. 91, no. 5, pp. 1683–90.

36 SR Davis, P McCloud, BJ Strauss and H Burger (1995) 'Testosterone enhances estradiol's effects on postmenopausal bone density and sexuality', *Maturitas*, vol. 21, pp. 227–36.

37 SR Davis et al (2008) 'Testosterone for low libido in postmenopausal women not taking estrogen', *The New England Journal of Medicine*, vol. 359, no. 19, pp. 2005–17.

38 Davis and Nijland, 'Pharmacological therapy for female sexual dysfunction', pp. 259–64.

39 ibid.; SL Davison et al (2005) 'Androgen levels in adult females: changes with age, menopause, and oophorectomy', *The Journal of Clinical Endocrinology & Metabolism*, vol. 90, no. 7, pp. 3847–53.

40 SR Davis et al (2005) 'Circulating androgen levels and self-reported sexual function in women', *JAMA*, vol. 294, no. 1, pp. 91–6.

41 SR Davis et al (2008) 'Testosterone for low libido in postmenopausal women not taking estrogen', *The New England Journal of Medicine*, vol. 359, no. 19, pp. 2005–17.

42 BioSante Pharmaceuticals (2011) 'LibiGel' <www.biosantepharma.com/LibiGel.php> [accessed November 2011].

43 SR Davis et al (2008) 'Testosterone for low libido in postmenopausal women not taking estrogen', *The New England Journal of Medicine*, vol. 359, no. 19, pp. 2005–17.

44 ME Wierman et al (2010) 'Endocrine aspects of women's sexual function', *Journal of Sexual Medicine*, vol. 7, pp. 561–85.

45 A Mason et al (2010) 'Sexual precocity in 4-year-old boy', *British Medical Journal*, vol. 340, no. 1, p. c2319 <www.bmj.com/content/340/bmj.c2319.full> [accessed 27 February 2011].

46 C Brachet et al (2005) 'Children's virilization and the use of a testosterone gel by their fathers', *European Journal of Pediatrics*, vol. 164, no. 10, pp. 646–7.

47 BGA Stuckey (2008) 'Female sexual function and dysfunction in the reproductive years: the influence of endogenous and exogenous sex hormones', *Journal of Sexual Medicine*, vol. 5, no. 10, pp. 2282–90.

48 A Davis and P Castaño (2006) 'Oral contraceptives and sexuality' in I Goldstein et al (eds), *Women's Sexual Function and Dysfunction: Study, diagnosis, and treatment*, Taylor and Francis, London and New York, pp. 290–6.

49 JL Shifren (2004) 'The role of androgens in Female Sexual Dysfunction', *Mayo Clinic Proceedings*, vol. 79, no. 4 suppl., pp. S19–24.

50 Davis and Nijland, 'Pharmacological therapy for female sexual dysfunction', pp. 259–64.

51 L Dennerstein, P Lehert and H Burger (2005) 'The relative effects of hormones and relationship factors on sexual function of women through natural menopause transition', *Fertility and Sterility*, vol. 84, pp. 174–80.

52 R Goldstat et al (2003) 'Transdermal testosterone improves mood, well being and sexual function in premenopausal women', *Menopause*, vol. 10, no. 5, pp. 390–8.

53 SR Davis et al (2008) 'Safety and efficacy of a testosterone metered-dose transdermal spray for treating decreased sexual satisfaction in premenopausal women: a randomized study', *Annals of Internal Medicine*, vol. 148, no. 6, pp. 569–77.

54 S Davis (2006) 'Available therapies and outcome results in premenopausal women' in I Goldstein et al (eds) *Women's Sexual Function and Dysfunction: Study, diagnosis, treatment*, Taylor & Francis, London and New York, pp. 539–48.

55 Recruitment for a 'Testosterone and Cognition Study (LIBIGEL STUDY)', Women's Health Research Program, Monash University, <www.med.monash.edu.au/medicine/alfred/womenshealth/participate/research-study.html> [accessed November 2011].

56 SR Davis and EA Nijland (2008) 'Pharmacological therapy for female sexual dysfunction: has progress been made?', *Drugs*, vol. 68, no. 3, pp. 259–64.

57 RA Lobo et al (2003) 'Comparative effects of oral esterified estrogens with and without methyltestosterone on endocrine profiles and dimensions of sexual function in postmenopausal women with hypoactive sexual desire', *Fertility and Sterility*, vol. 79, no. 6, pp. 1341–52.

58 C Pearson, A Allina and K Suthers (2006), an open letter to Andrew Von Eschenbach, Acting Commissioner US Food and Drug Administrator, 'Re: Citizen petition urging FDA to stop Solvay Pharmaceuticals and Breckenridge Pharmaceuticals from marketing esterified estrogens & methyltestosterone combination products', on behalf of the National Women's Health Network <www.fda.gov/ohrms/dockets/dockets/06p0346/06p-0346-cp00001–01-vol1.pdf> [accessed November 2011].

59 AJ Mohr (2009) 'The Rossbacher Law Firm, Hagens Berman Sobol Shapiro LLP, Wilentz Goldman & Spitzer, P.A., Reed Smith LLP and Thompson Hine LLP, announce the proposed settlement of a class action lawsuit concerning estratest and Solvay Pharmaceuticals, Inc.', *PR Newswire* <www.prnewswire.com/news-releases/the-rossbacher-law-firm-hagens-berman-sobol-shapiro-llp-wilentz-goldman--spitzer-pa-reed-smith-llp-and-thompson-hine-llp-announce-the-proposed-settlement-of-a-class-action-lawsuit-concerning-estratest-and-solvay-pharmaceuticals-inc-62019212.html> [accessed November 2011].

60 Pearson, Allina and Suthers, an open letter to Andrew Von Eschenbach, <www.fda.gov/ohrms/dockets/dockets/06p0346/06p-0346-cp00001–01-vol1.pdf. >.

61 Minutes of a meeting of the Advisory Committee for Reproductive Health Drugs (2004), U.S. Department of Health and Human Services, 2 December, Gaithersburg, Maryland <www.fda.gov/ohrms/dockets/ac/04/transcripts/2004–4082T1.pdf> [accessed November 2011].

62 Mohr, 'The Rossbacher Law Firm, Hagens Berman Sobol Shapiro LLP, Wilentz Goldman & Spitzer, P.A., Reed Smith LLP and Thompson Hine LLP, announce the proposed settlement of a class

action lawsuit concerning estratest and Solvay Pharmaceuticals, Inc.'.

63 'Court distributes $8.9 million to women's health organizations, universities, and charities nationwide' (2011) *Business Wire*, 8 March <www.businesswire.com/news/home/20110308007212/en/Court-Distributes-8.9-Million-Womens-Health-Organizations> [accessed November 2011].

64 'Solvay Pharmaceuticals, Inc. to discontinue supplying Estratest® brand tablets to U.S. Market' (2009) press release, 10 March.

65 'Esterified estrogens and methyltestosterone tablets' (2011) bulletin, American Society of Health-System Pharmacists, 2 April <www.ashp.org/DrugShortages/Current/Bulletin.aspx?id=552> [accessed November 2011].

66 S Cummings et al (2008) 'The effects of tibolone in older postmenopausal women', *The New England Journal of Medicine*, vol. 359, pp. 797–8.

67 M Doren et al (2001) 'Differential effects of the androgen status of postmenopausal women treated with tibolone and continuous combined estradiol and norethindrone acetate replacement therapy', *Fertility and Sterility*, vol. 75, pp. 554–9.

68 Cummings, 'The effects of Tibolone in older postmenopausal women', pp. 797–8.

69 EA Nijland, W Weijmar Schultz and J Nathorst-Boos (2008) 'Tibolone and transdermal E2/NETA for the treatment of female sexual dysfunction in naturally menopausal women: results from a randomized active-controlled trial', *Journal of Sexual Medicine*, vol. 5, pp. 646–56.

70 ME Wierman et al (2010) 'Endocrine aspects of women's sexual function', *Journal of Sexual Medicine*, vol. 7, pp. 561–85.

71 SR Davis and EA Nijland (2008) 'Pharmacological therapy for female sexual dysfunction: has progress been made?', *Drugs*, vol. 68, no. 3, pp. 259–64.

72 W Arlt et al (1999) 'Dehydroepiandrosterone replacement in women with adrenal insufficiency', *The New England Journal of Medicine*, vol. 341, no. 14, pp. 1013–20; EE Baulieu et al (2000) 'Dehydroepiandrosterone (DHEA), DHEA sulfate, and aging: contribution of the DHEAge Study to a sociobiomedical issue', Proceedings of the National Academy of Sciences of the United

States of America, vol. 97, no. 8, pp. 4279–84; AM Brooke et al (2006) 'Dehydroepiandrosterone improves psychological well-being in male and female hypopituity patients on maintenance growth hormone replacement', *Journal of Clinical Endocrinology & Metabolism*, vol. 91, no. 10, pp. 3773–9; F Labrie et al (2009) 'Effect of intravaginal dehydroepiandrosterone (Prasterone) on libido and sexual dysfunction in postmenopausal women', *Menopause*, vol. 16, no. 5, pp. 1–9; R Munarriz et al (2002) 'Androgen replacement therapy with dehydroepiandrosterone for androgen insufficiency and female sexual dysfunction: androgen and questionnaire results', *Journal of Sex & Marital Therapy*, vol. 28, no. Suppl 1, pp. 165–73.

73 SR Davis, M Panjari and FZ Stanczyk (2011) 'Clinical review: DHEA replacement for postmenopausal women', *Journal of Clinical Endocrinology & Metabolism*, vol. 96, no. 6, pp. 1642–53.

74 ME Wierman et al (2010) 'Endocrine aspects of women's sexual function', *Journal of Sexual Medicine*, vol. 7, pp. 561–85.

75 D Kritz-Silverstein et al (2008) 'Effects of Dehydroepiandrosterone Supplementation on cognitive function and quality of life: the DHEA and Well-Ness (DAWN) trial', *The American Geriatrics Society*, vol. 56, no. 7, pp. 1292–8.

76 K Delafrange (2007) 'Ladies "Viagra(r)" on the horizon', *G+*, <www.gplus.com/OBGYN/Insight/LADIES-VIAGRA-r-ON-THE-HORIZON-11090/> [accessed 2 November 2011].

77 L Crenshaw et al (1987) 'Pharmacologic modification of psychosexual dysfunction', *Journal of Sex & Marital Therapy*, vol. 13, no. 4, pp. 239–52.

78 RT Segraves et al (2001) 'Bupropion sustained release (SR) for the treatment of hypoactive sexual desire disorder (HSDD) in nondepressed women', *Journal of Sex & Marital Therapy*, vol. 27, no. 3, pp. 303–16; RT Segraves et al (2004) 'Bupropion sustained release for the treatment of hypoactive sexual desire disorder in premenopausal women', *Journal of Clinical Psychopharmacology*, vol. 24, no. 3, pp. 339–42.

79 JG Modell et al (2000) 'Effect of bupropion-SR on orgasmic dysfunction in nondepressed subjects: a pilot study', *Journal of Sex & Marital Therapy*, vol. 26, no. 3, pp. 231–40.

80 H Wessells quoted in D Rutz (1999) 'Tanning drug may find new life as Viagra alternative', *CNN*, <http://edition.cnn.com/HEALTH/men/9906/17/viagra.alternative/> [accessed 27 February 2011].

81 H Wessells et al (1998) 'Synthetic melanotropic peptide initiates erections in men with psychogenic erectile dysfunction: double-blind, placebo controlled crossover study', *Journal of Urology*, vol. 160, no. 2, pp. 389–93.

82 H Wessells et al (2000) 'Melanocortin receptor agonists, penile erection, and sexual motivation: human studies with Melanotan II', *International Journal of Impotence Research*, vol. 12, no. Suppl 4, pp. S74–9.

83 JG Pfaus et al (2004) 'Selective facilitation of sexual solicitation in the female rat by a melanocortin receptor agonist', Proceedings of the National Academy of Sciences of the United States of America, vol. 101, no. 27, pp. 10,201–4.

84 LE Diamond et al (2006) 'An effect on the subjective sexual response in premenopausal women with Sexual Arousal Disorder by Bremelanotide (PT–141), a melanocortin receptor agonist', *Journal of Sexual Medicine*, vol. 3, pp. 628–38.

85 L Tiefer quoted in J Dibbell (2006) 'Let us spray', *The Guardian* <www.guardian.co.uk/science/2006/apr/23/medicineandhealth.observermagazine> [accessed 2 November 2011].

86 I Goldstein et al (2006) *Women's Sexual Function and Dysfunction: Study, diagnosis and treatment*, Taylor & Francis, London and New York, p. 747.

Chapter 10

1 L Beitzig (1989) 'Causes of conjugal dissolution: a cross-cultural study', *Current Anthropology*, vol. 30, pp. 654–76.

2 A Vangelisti and M Gerstenberger (2004) 'Communication and marital infidelity' in J Duncombe et al (eds), *The state of affairs: explorations of infidelity and commitment*, Lawrence Erlbaum Associates, Mahway, NJ, pp. 59–79; B Buunk and P Dijkstra (2004) 'Men, women, and infidelity: sex differences in extradyadic sex and jealousy', in J Duncombe et al (eds) *The State of Affairs: Explorations of infidelity and commitment*, Lawrence Erlbaum Associates, Mahwey, NJ, p. 105.

3   A Brauer and D Brauer (1983) *ESO: How you and your lover can give each other hours of extended sexual orgasm*, Warner Books, New York.

4   D Schnarch (1997) *Passionate Marriage: Keeping love and intimacy alive in committed relationships*, Scribe, Melbourne, p. 227.

5   A Aron and E Aron (1986) *Love and the Expansion of Self: Understanding attraction and satisfaction*, Hemisphere, New York.

6   E Perel (2007) *Mating in Captivity: Sex, lies and domestic bliss*, Hodder & Stoughton, London.

7   J Morin (1995) *The Erotic Mind: Unlocking the inner sources of sexual passion and fulfilment*, HarperCollins, New York.

8   Brauer and Brauer, *ESO: How you and your lover can give each other hours of extended sexual orgasm*.

9   N Mondaini et al (2009) 'Regular moderate intake of red wine is linked to a better women's sexual health', *Journal of Sexual Medicine*, vol. 6, no. 10, pp. 2772–7.

10 C Fruteaua et al (2009) 'Supply and demand determine the market value of food providers in wild vervet monkeys', Proceedings of the National Academy of Sciences of the United States of America, vol. 106, no. 29, pp. 12007–12.

Conclusion

1   D Ackerman (1990) *A Natural History of the Senses*, postscript, Random House, New York.

Index

306.7082 ELL

Ellwood-Clayton, Bella.

Sex drive

JUL 1 6 2013